# ASSIGNMENT:
# TRUSTING GOD

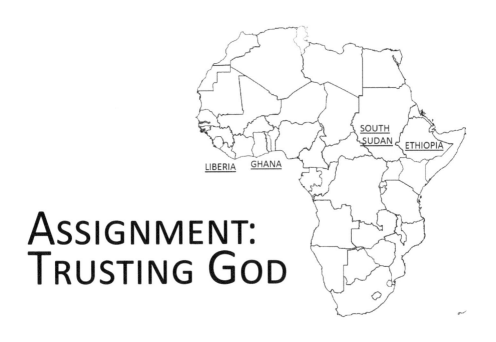

# ASSIGNMENT: TRUSTING GOD

## MEMOIRS OF MY ADVENTURES IN AFRICA
by Barb Hartwig

XULON PRESS

Xulon Press
2301 Lucien Way #415
Maitland, FL 32751
407.339.4217
www.xulonpress.com

Unless otherwise indicated,Scripture quotations taken from the New American Standard Bible (NASB). Copyright © 1960, 1962, 1963, 1968, 1971, 1972, 1973, 1975, 1977, 1995 by The Lockman Foundation. Used by permission. All rights reserved.

Printed in the United States of America.

ISBN-13: 9781545622780

To my nieces and nephews:
Chad, Mike, Misty, Kyle, Rachel, Tyler, and Briana.
May your lives be touched with these memoirs from Aunt Barb!

# ACKNOWLEDGMENTS

I cannot adequately thank Hadley Community Church, for their faithful support these thirty years and beyond; having assisted with the self-publishing of these memoirs. This story is yours and mine.

And I want to thank those who read and edited the early drafts of these memoirs: Steve and Jessica, Marge, Kristin, Ruth, Kent and Reta, and Elaine. Thank you so much.

# TABLE OF CONTENTS

# Glossary Of Abbreviations

**AIDS**—Acquired Immune Deficiency Syndrome caused by the HIV
**AIM**—Africa Inland Mission
**BCA**—Bible Church of Africa (Ghana)
**BELC**—Basic Education Learning Center
**BHSN**—Butterworth Hospital School of Nursing
**BNI**—Bureau of National Investigation (Ghana)
**CBHC**—Community-Based Health Care
**CEF**—Child Evangelism Fellowship
**CGS**—Columbia Graduate School (of Bible and Missions)
**CHW**—Community Health Worker
**CO**—Commanding Officer
**ELWA**—Eternal Love Winning Africa (Liberia)
**GMHC**—Global Missions Health Conference
**HIV**—Human Immunodeficiency Virus
**KHC**—Kale Heywet Church (translated to Word of Life, Ethiopia)
**9L1LP**—my Sierra Leone ham radio call sign
**NGO**—Non-Government Organization
**NPFL**—National Patriotic Front of Liberia
**PHC**—Primary Health Care
**RK**—Religious Knowledge (class)
**SIC**—Sudan Interior Church (Sudan)
**SIM**—formerly Sudan Interior Mission
**SL**—Sierra Leone
**SPLA**—Sudan People's Liberation Army
**TAR**—Traditional African Religion
**TBA**—Traditional Birth Attendant
**TEE**—Theological Education by Extension
**TTBA**—Trained Traditional Birth Attendant
**UN**—United Nation
**VHW**—Village Health Worker

# CHRONOLOGY

**1955**—Born at Goodrich Hospital, Michigan, USA

**1963**—Desire to be a missionary in Africa

**1967**—Accepted Jesus as my Savior

**1973**—Graduated from Lapeer High School

**1974**—Public commitment of my life to missionary work in Africa

**1976**—Graduated from Butterworth Hospital School of Nursing with diploma in nursing

**1977**—Short-term assignment with SIM at Bembereke Hospital, Benin, West Africa

**1978**—Graduated from Columbia Graduate School of Bible and Missions with diploma in Bible in Columbia, South Carolina

**1981**—Graduated from Goshen College in Goshen, Indiana with a Bachelor of Science in Nursing

**1982**—Attended SIM Candidate Orientation Course and was accepted as a member of SIM

**1983**—Assignment: Liberia for church planting and Community Based Health Care Program

*July 1990 "Detained at the border" of Liberia/Sierra Leone for eight days during Liberia's civil war (close call #1)

**1991–1992**—In Freetown, Sierra Leone, for Liberian refugee camp work and guesthouse manager for returnees to Liberia

**1993–1996**—Assignment: Ethiopia for administration; Metser Community Health; and then Makki Health station

*November 29, 1994—"Dodging bullets" at Metser station (close call #2)

**March 1996**—Visited Liberia for two weeks

**August 14–21, 1996**—Eight-day trip to Kenya to escort Ruth Clark home

**August 29, 1996**—My father died while I was home

**1997–2005**— Assignment: Ghana for church planting and Community Based Health Care Program

*February 28, 2004—"We are armed robbers" (close call #3) at my house in Tamale

**2006–2010** —Assignment: South Sudan
*April 26, 2008—"Plane crash" at Doro (close call #4)
**May 14, 2009**—My mother died while I was at Doro
**2011**—Assigned to the SIM Retirement Village Health office in Sebring, Florida and then furlough
**2012**—Assigned to Camp Barakel, Fairview, Michigan for one year
**February 28, 2013**— Resigned from SIM after 30 years of active service

---

*The four close calls in Africa

# INTRODUCTION

*The writing of* these memoirs is first and foremost a permanent record of God's faithfulness in the life of an ordinary person. A line in the song *Amazing Grace* says, "Through many dangers, toils, and snares, I have already come." I want to shout, "To God be the glory, great things He has done!" These accounts will not only record the facts at the urging of friends and family, but hopefully give balance to the dangers, toils, and snares I went through.

Highlighting my adventures in Africa—especially the four close calls God took me through—hopefully will inspire and challenge all who would follow Christ, from youth to old age. I laugh because more often than not, these close calls are what others remember about my career in Africa and not the health care and Bible teaching! It seems Community Based Health Care as a part of church planting is less and less common. I would encourage others to delve in and do it. I was not able to hand over my work to someone else in any of the places where I worked. Maybe this story will be my hand over and provide insight for others to choose Community Based Health Care as part of their life's path.

The following is a short, slightly edited excerpt from my September, 1990, prayer letter written about our harrowing exit from Liberia: "Up to this time Cape Mount County had been relatively trouble free. However, unknown to us, it was invaded by sea by the rebels on July 20 while we were at Tahn packing up to leave. When we reached the Sierra Leone border on July 21 to cross over, the Liberian government soldiers detained us for two days. They confiscated our U.S. passports and seized our two Land Cruisers. On Sunday July 22 at 5:30 in the afternoon, the rebels launched a surprise attack on the border post. We had made a barricade in the customs room and lay on the floor during the hour of shooting. We praise God for protecting us during that crucial and frightening hour of attack and that the rebels were helpful once we could identify ourselves. We still spent a week at a town about fifteen miles from the border. The Lord graciously sent one Southern Baptist missionary over to Liberia to help negotiate our release. On July 28, we walked out of Liberia empty-handed, but rejoicing to be safe, free, and alive!" After that experience I resolved to trust the Lord even more **no matter what**. I believe that what He does cannot be wrong, even if I don't understand. Have you had a **"no matter what"** experience in your life?

Once I was on a panel of three missionaries answering questions from my fellow South Sudan field missionaries. At the time, I had spent twenty-seven years pre-Africa and twenty-seven years on active assignment in Africa. They asked the panel what helped us stick it out serving the Lord cross-culturally for so long. My answer was these three things:

1. Guarding my daily quiet time with God in His Word.
2. Resilience: being willing to take another assignment when one ended. For example, I did not want to leave Liberia, but I had to, and I took another assignment in Africa.
3. Psalms 37:1 says, "Do not fret because of evil doers." Second Corinthians 4:8 says, "perplexed, but not despairing." Having the attitude "why should I be spared from trouble" helped me to cope and not fall into deep self-pity or depression.

Lord, I'm keeping my eyes on you: following you, Lord. I won't look to the left or right, keeping You in my sight.

# Part One
## Ready, Set, Go!

Hadley, Michigan

Lapeer High School, Michigan

Butterworth Hospital School of Nursing, Grand Rapids, Michigan

Bembereke Hospital, Benin, West Africa

Columbia Bible College, South Carolina

Goshen College, Indiana

SIM headquarters, Cedar Grove, New Jersey

Tahn, Liberia, West Africa

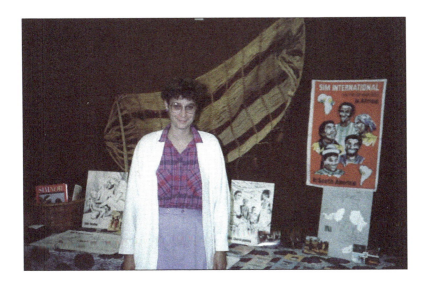

## CHAPTER 1

# My Early Life (1955–1973)

*God needs helpers* from every demographic, no matter location, age, rich, or poor. In my case, I was born in 1955 as the second-oldest daughter of a hard-working farmer. My great-grandfather, of German heritage, settled the farm in 1876, near the rural town of Hadley, Michigan. Both my parents, Gene and Beverly Hartwig, were Christians and took us four kids to town to attend the Hadley Community Church, which became my home church. To my knowledge, I am the first missionary in my family.

My father did not only have sixty cattle in the barn to feed morning and night; he also had a self-employed business laying drain tile. Using a machine, he would dig a trench and worked hard laying clay tiles end to end in a ditch through the fields for drainage. It was a big deal when Dad took his preschool children to work with him on occasion. Through my dad's example, I was self-motivated to get work done. That mattered because doing community health work is not the same as being on a shift schedule like a nurse in a clinic or hospital.

After the drainage tile years, Dad built a pole barn and expanded our beef cattle farming to 250 cattle. His shop was extensively supplied and equipped. He loved to fix things. He did not buy any new machinery. My parents had four children in seven years. Mom did the business and family accounting. She was also church treasurer, church organist, church Ladies Fellowship founder (first president), and managed to work as a bank teller for several years.

Grandma, Eva Elizabeth Jagow Potter, was very important in our lives. She helped my mother a lot. I was eight years old when I first knew I wanted to be a missionary in Africa. God put that desire in my heart one Sunday evening when SIM missionaries Winston and Mary Ellen Adams showed pictures of their work in Nigeria. Grandma was the first and only one I told initially about my desire to become a missionary. I remember standing at our kitchen counter as I explained to her what I planned to do when I grew up, and she believed me.

Besides Winston and Mary Ellen Adams, our Hadley Church supported Dr. Hal and Connie (Brigham) White as SIM missionaries to Nigeria. Connie grew up on the Brigham farm just a mile down the road from our farm. Connie was a playmate with my mother and my Aunt Lucy Potter because of the friendship between Eva Potter (my Grandma) and Connie's mother (Sarah Brigham). I'm sure Mom and Connie never dreamed as children that Mom would marry into the Hartwig family and live on Brigham Road one day. In the mid-1960s I was fascinated with the Lassa Fever discovery story coming out of Nigeria from Hal and Connie White. Dr. Hal was the only surviving doctor caring for Lassa victims at one point in time (see the book *Fever* for the whole story). The Lassa Fever outbreak is the reason I became interested in medical missions. In high school I also found an interest in emergency medicine. It was off to nursing school for me after graduating from Lapeer High School in 1973. See chapter 3 for a first-hand encounter I had with Lassa Fever on my short-term trip to Benin! This connection to SIM through the Adams and the Whites is what eventually drew me into SIM membership one day.

When I was about thirteen years old, I accepted Christ as my Savior. Everybody thought I had already done that, but I knew in my heart that it was not real until one Sunday evening service when a visiting preacher talked about Hell. I went forward to pray with him, confess my sin, and ask Jesus into my heart. It was real, and it felt so good to have that settled in my heart and mind! I remember the preacher saying, "For God so loved *Barb Hartwig* that He gave His only begotten Son . . .", from John 3:16 with my name added. About two years later, our youth group at church attended an evangelistic service, and I dedicated my life to Christ that night and promised to serve Him with all my heart as Lord of my life. I started having daily devotions and still do today. I believe daily Bible reading and prayer have sustained my faith through many difficult times.

In high school, my social life revolved all around our youth group at church. I was not involved in after-school activities because we were farming, and we lived twelve miles from school. In retrospect, I would have liked to try out for track and field events. I liked to run. On Eighth-grade Field Day, I won the 100-yard dash and our team won the relay race. That was a big deal for me, and I remember wishing my mother would have been there in the stands to see it. It was at this time that my parents expanded the beef cattle business, and it was work, work, and more work at home. They made it a point to instill a strong work ethic in all four of us kids.

In high school, I searched and prayed often to know God's will for my life. I thought I should have some undeniable sign from God that it was His call and His desire for me to serve as a missionary. I wanted to be a missionary in the worst way, but I got hung up on whether it was God's will. I had a Nehemiah type of call (Lord, can I?), not the Jonah type (Lord, I don't want to go). Later on, in college, God settled in my mind His will that I was to proceed with cross-cultural missions. I learned that God guides us by His Word, prayer, circumstances, and the wise counsel of other Christians. Some common mistakes made by those seeking God's will are:

1. Do not think that because you want to do something, it cannot be the will of God.
2. Do not feel that every decision must have a bolt of confirmation. James 1:5 says to pray for wisdom and God will give it.
3. There are logical implications that fall into line, such as simply a desire in your heart for missions.
4. Avoid thinking you are in the will of God if everything is moonlight and roses. In Mark chapter four, the disciples obeyed and went to sea, yet the storm came. Expect trials and difficulties.
5. Avoid thinking a call to missionary service is different from the call to anything else.
6. Avoid thinking that if we fall into sin, we can never be used by God.
7. Avoid the temptation to sit and wait and do nothing.

My mother and grandma taught me to cook and bake. I like kitchen work and had lots of practice at home. Hospitality turned out to be one of my favorite things to do in Africa. I took up 4-H sewing, and Grandma taught me to quilt and mend, which also came in handy in Africa. I love to read books, and that served me well in Africa to fill those long evenings alone. Nothing I learned went in vain. All the hard work and basic skills I learned at home on the farm would come in very useful in Africa. Even knowing how to ride a horse was useful when I got to Ethiopia and rode a white mule named Ozzie up the mountain to visit a village. I also believe that my farm life resulted in a strong immune system, because I did not get sick very often in Africa.

Money in our family was tight. This too was a good lesson for missionary work. I did a lot of babysitting to buy material and make my own clothes. When my older sister, Kathy, and I and our two younger brothers, Robert and Ken, were in grade school my parents gave us a cow. We named him Troubles. Sometimes, we put Kathy's saddle on him and rode him. Well, when Troubles was finally sold at market, we each opened up a savings account. The only thing we were allowed to do with that money was buy another calf. Each of us invested in another calf. And when each steer was sold, the money went into our savings account. After high school graduation, we could spend our savings any way we wanted to. My savings paid for my first year of tuition at Butterworth Hospital School of Nursing. My last steer was sold in my freshman year at Butterworth, and he (Frelly) paid for my entire second year of nursing school tuition. Thank God for the foresight of my parents to teach us to save. We worked hard on our farm and earned our savings. My father never handed out money to us kids. He was generous in many ways, but not with money.

I graduated from Lapeer High School in 1973. It was a big deal to leave home and start college two and a half hours drive away from home. Even then, I knew it was good to get used to being away from home. Leaving home never did get easier for me. I missed my family very much in college and in Africa. Nevertheless, God enabled me to be content and always look forward to my next time home, be that a matter of weeks or years. Yes, preparation for the mission field started at home growing up. There was no pampering at our house, but we knew we were loved, and I thank God for my parents and sister and brothers.

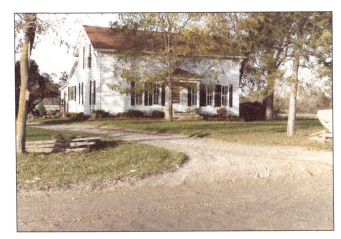

Hartwig's family home

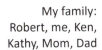

My family: Robert, me, Ken, Kathy, Mom, Dad

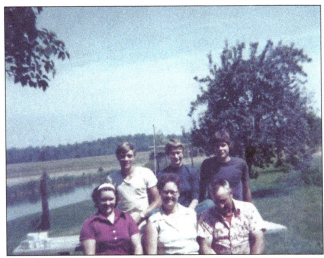

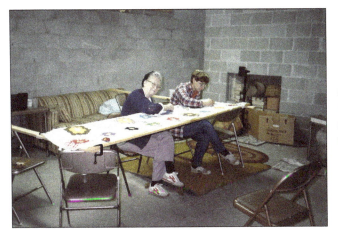

Grandma Potter and I, sewing and talking for hours!

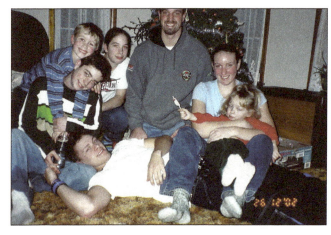

My seven nieces
and nephews

I thank God for all I
learned by growing
up on a farm.

Kathy, Robert,
Ken and I.

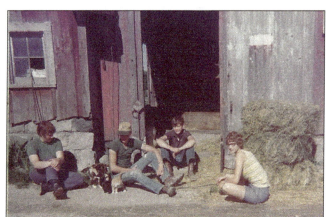

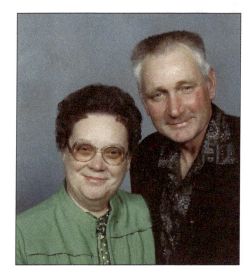

My parents,
Gene and
Beverly Hartwig

## CHAPTER 2

# COLLEGE YEARS (1973–1981)

*It took me* nine years to complete my college education and work to pay for it. I was jumping through all the hoops necessary to prepare for a career on the mission field. Three times I graduated from a college program. After I passed the Michigan State Boards in nursing in 1976, I worked as a Registered Nurse either part-time or full-time in various hospitals. I gained nursing experience in the coronary care unit, surgical ward, emergency room nursing, and orthopedics. I earned the pocket money I needed to live on and paid for my college tuition. In retrospect, I could have applied for grants or scholarships, but I didn't know how to do that.

**Butterworth Hospital School of Nursing (BHSN)**

At BHSN in Grand Rapids, Michigan, I grew up. I was naïve about many things when I arrived there at the age of seventeen. It was hard, but, praise the Lord, I studied hard, enjoyed friendships, learned to live away from home, and I did not miss a single day of attendance in those three years of nursing school.

During my second year at Butterworth in 1974, I attended the Calvary Church Missions Conference. This was the Church on Michigan Avenue where Rev. Gardner was the minister. Mr. Rudy Nilson from SIM was a speaker at the conference, and one night after he preached, he gave an altar call for anyone willing to commit to serve God as a missionary. I went forward and prayed with him. That public commitment finalized my decision to be a missionary in Africa. I went back to the dorm and phoned my family and told them all about it. It was full steam ahead to missions after that, and everyone knew that was my goal. My roommate, Karen Cleary, was also committed to the mission field, and we supported each other in many ways. We enjoyed the Nurses Christian Fellowship group at Butterworth those three years.

My good friend Gwen Pinter and I remain friends to this day. And my "big sister" Jean Harvey Perdue, from the class ahead of us, has also been my good friend and supporter throughout my years in SIM. Jean sent me innumerable packages throughout my years in Africa and even came to visit me in Liberia in 1989.

Butterworth's nursing program gave each of us a diploma in nursing. All of our written tests were given in multiple choice format in preparation for State Boards. This resulted in all sixty-six of us from the class of 1976 passing State Boards the first time around. It is unfortunate, in my opinion, that stand-alone hospital nursing diploma programs were closed down in favor of college or university programs alone. I thank God for the practical experience I received at Butterworth before graduating.

After graduation from Butterworth, I moved back home and worked in the Coronary Care unit at McLaren Hospital in Flint, Michigan, for one year. They granted me a three-month leave of absence in 1977 to do a short-term mission assignment in Benin, West Africa.

## Columbia Graduate School of Bible and Missions (CGS)

My favorite year of college was at Columbia Graduate School of Bible and Missions in Columbia, South Carolina. I loved studying Bible and met some really good friends there. This diploma in Bible program only lasted from September 1977 to June 1978.

I remember that a group of fellow classmates threw a surprise birthday party for me! I must have turned twenty-two years old that fall. It was a socially good year for me. The combination of good friends and studying the Bible was a lot of fun during that time of my life. In my opinion, every Christian should "do" at least one year at a Bible College.

My sister's wedding took place in October of 1977. I flew home for the weekend. Kathy and Barry had a lovely wedding at our home church in Hadley and a reception at the Hadley town hall. She even made her own wedding dress. The wedding was on Friday night in Hadley, and then Barry's family had a reception for them in Scottville on Saturday night. They had a polka band. It was expected that the wedding party take the first dance. I was really nervous because I had never danced before, and I had signed a pledge with Columbia

Bible College that I would not dance while a student. Yet, somehow, I did it with Barry's brother, the best man. I almost missed my flight back to Columbia because my brother Robert went hunting on Sunday, and we left late from Scottville. He did not calculate that I had to go home to Hadley first and get my suitcase before we could drive to the Detroit airport!

While at Bible College I made a decision. I made a personal commitment that I would be a "package deal." That is, I would not date a guy who was not also committed to being a missionary as well. It was me AND missions. I lived in a module on campus with several other girls and our "mod mom" was Elaine. Elaine and Burt Haaga got married and eventually joined SIM, and served the Lord in Niger for about thirty years.

Many mission organizations came to Columbia Bible College to recruit. I looked around, but decided to go with SIM. That was no small final decision either. The peace I felt with that decision was the Holy Spirit confirming it was the right one.

While at Bible College, I worked every other weekend at Columbia Presbyterian Hospital in downtown Columbia in the Emergency Room. It was both challenging and fun. It gave me some spending money. My little Ford Pinto car served me well for several years. I did not have enough money saved up to pay my tuition for that year. My brother Robert lent me what I lacked to pay tuition, room, and board. I paid him back as soon as I could.

June 1978 included a whirlwind of a week as I took final exams and drove home just in time for my brother Ken's high school graduation open house. If I remember right, his open house was on a Sunday afternoon, and I had to report for work at Spring Hill Camps as summer camp nurse that very same evening. My good friend Gwen Pinter flew down to Columbia and helped me drive home. To this day, I do not like long car trips and certainly not by myself. I never unpacked my car from Bible College that Sunday. I needed everything for the summer at Spring Hill Camps in Evart, Michigan. I had almost no money for the summer. About all I could afford was some gas money to occasionally go home for a weekend. I will never forget that Robert once handed me money to go buy a pair of jeans that summer. It about gives me tears to think of it now.

After three months of hard work as a camp nurse in 1978, the camp paid me $500. Most of that went to pay my car insurance. I went back to McLaren Hospital in Flint, Michigan, to work for one year. This time I worked as a team leader on a large surgical ward. It was a difficult job because we were understaffed most evenings. The upside of work that year was establishing lasting friendships with two colleagues named Kristin Lewis and Peggy Benson. We have made many vacation trips together over the years since, and I often thank God for their true friendship and support. Living at home that year enabled me to pay off Bible College debts and save for Goshen College tuition.

## Goshen College

From August 1979 to April 1981, I was one of nine Registered Nurse students in a Nursing Bachelor of Science (BSN) course in Goshen, Indiana. I liked the Amish and Mennonite community around Goshen. I liked living off campus at a house with four bedrooms rented out to college students. Miriam Hostetler was in charge of the house and became my best friend at Goshen. Unfortunately, I did not care for the college course. However, I completed it for my degree in nursing. I worked three or four days a week at Goshen Hospital to pay my way through. This degree did prove important in applying for long-term work permits in Africa.

As I finished up the degree requirements, I felt the time to leave for a career in Africa growing closer and closer, and that excited me so much! God had truly put a desire in my heart for the people in Africa. I was anxious to move on!

The most interesting class I took at Goshen was an elective class in Hansens Disease (Leprosy) at Carville, Louisiana. Our instructor, Kay Yutzy, drove us down South for the three-week course. I learned a lot and met Dr. Paul Brand, who brilliantly pioneered research on the disease of leprosy in India. He was world renowned as a hand surgeon. Dr. Brand and Philip Yancey co-authored a book called *Fearfully and Wonderfully Made*, which I highly recommend as a refreshing look at the human and spiritual body.

Mom and Dad came to my graduation program at Goshen and took home all my "stuff" with them because a group of us girls had signed up for a week-long bike trip in Florida. We drove my car to the panhandle of Florida, leaving the evening after commencement and drove all night. We rode about thirty miles a day in a group of around twenty. Bikes were provided. I had had no practice. It was all right until the last day when we encountered some hills. I had to walk my bike a couple of times. It was fun, but I was sore and tired.

Finally, my college years were done. After the bike trip, I went home for another year and worked at McLaren Hospital in Flint again. This time I worked evenings on the orthopedic floor as a team leader. I did it, but I also knew even then that hospital work was not for me! McLaren Hospital granted me another leave of absence. This time it was to attend SIM's one-month candidate school for membership into the mission! Hurrah! No doubts on my part. I was totally on board with this commitment. Little did I imagine how I had yet to really learn to trust God—no matter what. So far in life I had got to do everything I wanted to do.

CHAPTER 3

# SHORT TERM TRIP TO BENIN, WEST AFRICA (1977)

*In between nursing* school and Bible college, I went to Africa for three months. In December 1976, I attended Intervarsity's Urbana Missionary Conference in order to meet SIM representatives there. I already knew God's call on my life and wanted to discuss future steps I needed to take. They advised me to "do" a short-term mission trip. I was very excited about this opportunity.

McLaren Hospital granted me a leave of absence between March and June of 1977. My home church, Hadley Community Church, raised the funds I needed to go. My parents drove me to JFK airport in New York City. It was tough leaving them. I was almost twenty-one years old. But once in the air, I felt the freedom and excitement of following God's will to Africa. It was my first time on a plane.

Bembereke Hospital in Benin operates in the French language. I did not know French. This huge barrier drove home to me the importance of language learning. I vowed never to return to a Francophone country to work without learning French. Another big decision I made after this short-term assignment was that I did not want to be assigned to a mission hospital. Bembereke scheduled me to work all different shifts. Even if I could have spoken the language, my schedule would have prevented me from having even a Children's Bible Club. This short-term opportunity was very important because I learned what I did NOT want to do when I came back to Africa to serve in a long-term capacity! In the years to come, I counseled many a short-termer to look around and see what everyone was doing. Even if one does not like their short-term assignment, see what would spark a passion! That's what happened to me.

Getting away from the hospital compound was not possible very often, but I really enjoyed the local market, the local church, a nearby

Bariba village, and one trip to Parakou town. Snakes, scorpions, coping with the heat, having little meat or cheese, a severe water shortage in May, the language barrier, homesickness, etc., were challenges. Ruth Wetmore from South Africa was the head nurse at the hospital, and she opened up her home to me those three months. I still remember the evening Ruth and I roasted miniature marshmallows over candle light for our dessert! We enjoyed sharing the cooking and baking. I learned so much from Ruth during that time.

Carol Guth was an American nurse working in the outpatient department of Bembereke. She advised me to get my BS degree in nursing. That would be another important decision I made based on this short-term service. This experience in Africa helped me settle down to finish my education and be prepared for long-term service. One cannot join SIM with any financial debt, so I had to work and pay off my college debts before attending the SIM candidate course.

Four things happened toward the end of my three months in Benin, which must be recorded.

1. One week before I was to leave Benin, our SIM hospital lab technician, Elsbeth Lenherr, from Switzerland, fell very sick. She was unconscious. The missionary doctors diagnosed hepatitis. They decided to evacuate her to our SIM Hospital in Nigeria. Because I lived with the matron of nurses, Ruth Wetmore, I assisted with Elsbeth's evacuation. They laid her on my army cot (which I had slept on for three months), and at daybreak we put her in a vehicle and drove her to the border of Nigeria, where, by a miracle, our communications worked and she was met by SIMers on the Nigeria side. They took her to the mission hospital, but Elsbeth died the next day. An autopsy report revealed weeks later that she died from Lassa Fever! She must have picked it up in the lab. It is a miracle that there was no outbreak of Lassa. It is a very contagious virus and very deadly, much like Ebola.

2. On my second-to-last night at Bembereke, while Ruth and I were asleep, robbers broke into our house at night and stole many things, including my purse with passport and money in it. In fact, they broke into four houses that night on the hospital

compound. Ruth and I were not awakened during the robbery. The local people said there is an incense that can be burned outside one's bedroom window through the screen that puts one into a deeper sleep. Maybe the robbers used it. I could not travel without my passport, so we prayed. The next day my purse was found shaken out with all contents, minus the money, on the mountainside behind our house! My passport was there! Praise the Lord. I was able to leave as scheduled the next day to go to Nigeria and visit Winston and Mary Ellen Adams.

3. After farewells at Bembereke, friends drove me to the Nigeria border, where I crossed and flew by SIM AIR to Kano in Northern Nigeria. I spent a week with our church missionaries, Winston and Mary Ellen Adams. He was the one who spoke at our church the night I felt called to be a missionary at the age of eight. What a special week I had with them! Winston and Mary Ellen were at an agricultural school for orphan boys in a small village called Roni in the Islamic northern region of Nigeria. I remember a severe sand storm blowing in one night off the Sahara Desert. Wow! Everything was covered with Sahara sand despite closing up the houses as tight as we could. This visit was important because the next year, 1978, our beloved missionary Winston Adams became critically ill. Despite being evacuated to England, he died. Mary Ellen and her three children returned to Nigeria and continued ministering at the boarding school for missionary children. My home church continued to support Mary Ellen and does so even today in her retirement. I call Mary Ellen my "SIM mom".

4. I was booked to leave Nigeria on SIM's last charter plane out of Nigeria. Everyone on board was with SIM. I happened to sit next to Penny Pinneo, the first survivor of Lassa Fever back in 1965. I knew of her by reputation. What a privilege to speak with her on that flight home. If I had known then that Elsbeth had died of Lassa Fever, it would have been an even more interesting conversation on our way home!

The subject of Lassa was not over. My first day at home I had a surprise visit from our county health department nurse explaining that a person on our flight was very sick, and they suspected Lassa Fever. Everyone on that flight was warned and had to take their temperature every day and report any fever or symptoms. It later turned out that the sick child on our flight did not have Lassa Fever. Little did we know how close I HAD been to a real Lassa case just about two weeks before the chartered flight home!

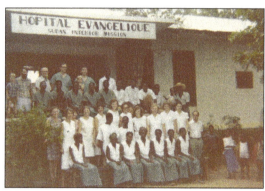

Staff at Bembereke
Hospital in
Benin, West Africa, 1977.
I am the second
nurse standing
from the right side
of that row.

I did hospital work for
three months on my
short-term assignment
at Bembereke Hospital.

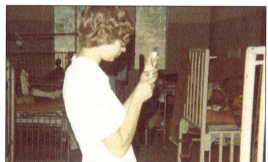

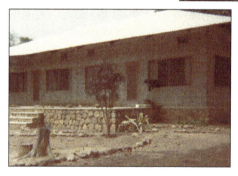

This is a duplex on the
hospital compound.
Ruth Wetmore shared her home with
me, on the right side of this duplex.
I slept on an armycot just inside and
below the front window

Article in *Africa Now* magazine,
Sudan Interior Mission,
January-February 1978

### SIMer dies of Lassa Fever

CEDAR GROVE, NJ (SIM) — SIM has lost its third missionary to Lassa Fever. While working at Bimbereke Hospital in Benin Republic, lab technician Elsbeth Lenherr of Switzerland came down with what was diagnosed as hepatitis. A week later she was flown to Jos, where she died the next day.

Although symptoms did not match those usually associated with Lassa Fever, blood tests were conducted at the National Communicable Diseases Center in Atlanta, Georgia, and "proved conclusively" that the cause of death was indeed the dread virus. Hers is the first proven death from Lassa Fever in Benin.

The first victim in SIM was nurse Charlotte Shaw, who died in 1968, when Lassa Fever was first identified. One year later, Dr. Jeanette Troup died. Blood from survivor Lily Pinneo has since been a source of serum for treating victims.

CHAPTER 4

# CANDIDATE ORIENTATION AND DEPUTATION (1982)

*If my college* years were the "Get Ready," then deputation is the "Get Set."

In April of 1982 I went to SIM USA headquarters in Cedar Grove, New Jersey. I had been invited to SIM Candidate School after completing many required steps. Candidate orientation would be a four-week opportunity for each candidate and the mission to get to know each other. It culminated in each candidate for membership meeting individually with the SIM USA Board for an extensive interview.

The SIM call letters originally stood for Sudan Interior Mission. Back in 1893 when the Mission began, "Sudan" was the sub-Sahara territory of Africa stretching from Liberia on the Atlantic coast to the country of Sudan on the east. The region of the Soudan (not misspelled) is marked as such on the old map of Africa I have had on the wall above my desk at home since college. This old Africa map is featured on the front cover of these memoirs. In 1982 a South American mission merged into S.I.M., so they broadened the letters of S.I.M. to stand for Society of International Ministries. S.I.M. changed again many years later to stand for Serving In Mission. Today the letters SIM (without periods) stand alone as the name of this international, interdenominational church-planting mission. But, of course, we insiders say it stands for "Sure I'll Move!"

My college debts were paid, my higher education completed, and my passion for missions never higher. God was at work in my life, and the cross-cultural adventure with God was really starting. Our first night upon arriving at candidate "school," we met together with the SIM USA director, Mr. Trevor Ardill. I distinctly remember the solemn words he said to us. He read Philippians 2:13: "For it is God which worketh in you both to will and to do of his good pleasure." And then Mr. Ardill said, "Anyone here who is not sure that God has called you to this work of missions should turn around and go home." Yes, that simple. You could have heard a pin drop. I knew in my heart that God had called me and given me a charge to fulfill the Great Commission by going to Africa. I stayed. And so did the other twenty or so candidates.

Let me quote from Helen Roseveare's book *Give Me This Mountain:* "If you think you have come to the mission field because you are a little better than others, or as the cream of your church, or because of your medical degree, or for the service you can render the African Church, or even for the souls you may see saved, you will fail. Remember, the Lord has only one purpose ultimately for each one of us, to make us more like Jesus. He is interested in your relationship with Himself. Let Him take you and mold you as He will; all the rest will take its rightful place."

In Deuteronomy Joshua and Caleb looked at the human odds, but said, we have a big God. In Joshua 1:7 it is written, "Be strong and courageous." After reading Hudson Taylor's biography, Helen Roseveare's books, Isobel Kuhn's books, and many other missionary accounts, I knew that what Mr. Ardill said was true. If one is afraid or unsure, go home. The road ahead will not be easy.

In about the second week of candidate orientation, each prospective missionary was to meet individually with the candidate committee. I was a bit nervous and intimidated by this committee, which consisted of all men, even before my turn came. When I was called in, Mr. Ardill said to me, "What if I was an African and asked you, 'Why should I believe in your God?' What would you say?" I stumbled through an answer, and when I finally left them, I really thought I was done for. When Phyllis Lloyd found out what it was like "in there" for me, she stepped in and from then on was on that committee and helped support the other women candidates. I do not know what all she said to the committee, but I think it was less intimidating for the others.

Jessica Layman was another single candidate in the April 1982 class. She is from South Bend, Indiana. We quickly became friends. Before leaving candidate school, each candidate was to have selected their field assignment and do a presentation on the country they were going to. I was the last one to get an assignment because all the openings for nurses were either at a hospital or clinic. I explained that after my short-term at Bembereke, God was leading me into something else. I said, "For example, what I see Joy Crombie is doing in Liberia." Long story short, SIM's International Personnel Director, Mr. Hedley Waldock, got on the ham radio to Liberia and asked if Joy needed any help. The answer came back "yes." I was thrilled. I accepted the opportunity to work on a church-planting team in this English-speaking country. And it just so happened that Jessica was going to Liberia too! We immediately made plans to go out together on the same flight, and that is exactly what we did. Meeting the SIM USA Board on our final day was a breeze. They had a few questions for me, and I left Cedar Grove a member of SIM.

Having a solid membership in a local church is a big step forward for any missionary raising the prayer and financial support needed to work cross-culturally, a process known as deputation. Hadley Community Church was prepared to support me in missions ever since my commitment in 1974. My home church promised to give 50% of whatever my support requirement was for the duration of my career! That is no small commitment. When I started out in 1983, I needed $770 per month of pledged support. Thirty years later in 2013 I needed $2,500 a month, and my home church kept its promise to give half of that amount all that time. God bless their faithfulness to God and me.

I must relay a phone call I received from Pastor Peter DeKlerk at Hunters Creek Community Church (HCCC) in December, 1982. This church is only ten miles away from Hadley. He said they would pick up whatever amount I was lacking in pledged support. And he did not ask or know what I was lacking. I will never forget that. It turned out to be only $25 per month then. But it enabled me to tell SIM that I was fully supported and ready to go. In the years that followed, HCCC increased their monthly support considerably. Pastor Peter and Norma DeKlerk were SIM Ethiopia missionary alumni. Pastor Peter answered almost every prayer letter I wrote with a personal note, which I highly appreciated over the years. I also want to add that my cousin Mike and Sue Hartwig introduced me to Lovells Chapel in the Grayling, Michigan, area up north. Lovells Chapel committed to my support for the whole thirty years too. So I had three churches and about twenty-four individuals who faithfully supported me. Most of them did so for my whole missionary career! In my last five years with SIM, Calvary Bible Church in Lapeer, Michigan, supported me too.

I will quote from the March-April, 1988 issue of *SIM NOW* magazine, "Yonder . . . is a gold mine. I will descend and dig, but you at home must hold the ropes" (William Carey). Picture the missionary descending a rope into a mine or well and the Church is holding the rope. We, that is, missionaries, do require the prayers and financial assistance of many to be able to go and serve overseas.

A bit of advice to prospective missionaries: maintain a strong home church affiliation and talk with them about your calling and plans, and, secondly, keep in touch with your supporters regularly. That is, beyond the prayer letters that go out three or four times a year; hand-written notes and acknowledgments mean the most. It will go a long way to sustaining their interest and commitment. Do not depend on social media to substitute for personal communication with your supporters. Also, do not expect your supporters to write to you. Most probably will not, but just keep on writing to them.

Remember, there is no Go without the Lo! In Matthew 28:19, 20 Jesus said, "Go therefore and make disciples of all the nations . . . and lo, I am with you always, even to the end of the age." On January 9, 1983, my church held a commissioning service for me. Mr. Fred Zabel, SIM's regional director, gave the commissioning message and charge. Pastor Bruce Craner gave the charge to the church to support me. My friend Miriam Hostetler, accompanied by her mother, from Goshen, Indiana, came and sang two special songs that night. They were *"Christ Means More to Me Than Anything"* and *"So Send I You."* What a meaningful night for everyone there. I have put a copy of my commissioning service program at the end of this chapter. Despite my tears, I was happy and ready to make the break with my family and home country.

God did test my zeal and determination over the thirty years that I would be on assignment in Africa and a member of SIM. I recall that I signed up for a one credit volleyball course at Goshen College. I got halfway through it and quit. It was the only time I dropped out of a course I started. I quit because I found myself hoping the ball would not come to me. I was afraid I would miss it or not do the right thing (bump, set, strike). I compared myself to others. While later reflecting back on that, I learned an important life principle. I learned that I should have wanted the ball to come to me in order to learn. James 1:25 says to become an effectual doer of the Word we must face trials with joy. I had no idea about the dangerous close calls, the civil war upheaval, burying three missionaries, etc., that would be the reality of my life as a missionary. But I was not going to only read about the mission field and the Great Commission and spiritual needs, but go and do something about it. Give me the ball. I would take a calculated risk and go for it with God beside me all the way. For there is no Go without the Lo!

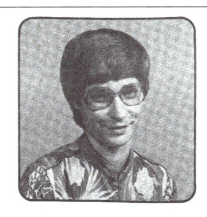

New in
**SIM**

Barb Hartwig

Since childhood Barb has felt God's leading in her life to be involved in medical miss-ions. This was confirmed through a short term of service with the SIM in 1977 at the Bembereke Hospital in Benin. Barb is a reg-istered nurse and has graduated from the Columbia Graduate School of Bible and Missions.

Barb's interests are in Bible study groups and village health care. She has been appointed to missionary service with the SIM in Liberia.

Needs:
Preparatory:
    1. Initial air fare and freight    $1700
    2. Initial outfit and equipment    1000

On-going:
    1. Prayer partners to faithfully stand
       with her
    2. Monthly support    $770

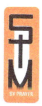

Barb Hartwig
4884 Brigham Road
Goodrich, MI 48438

**SUDAN INTERIOR MISSION □ Cedar Grove, NJ 07009**

MISSIONARY COMMISSIONING SERVICE
Barb Hartwig
ELWA-Box 192
Monrovia, Liberia
January 9, 1983

Hymn 483    "We've a Story to Tell"

Invocation    Kent Copeman

Scripture Reading    First Commissioning
Acts 13:1-5
Phil. 1:20-2:5    Paul's Expectations

Presentation of Missionary and Missionary Testimony

Special    "Christ Means More to Me Than Anything"
Mim Hostetler, friend from Goshen, IN

Commissioning Message    Rev. Fred Zabel
                         SIM Regional Rep.

Charge to Missionary    Rev. Fred Zabel

Charge to Church    Pastor Cramer

Commissioning Prayer    Pastor Cramer

Presentation of Commissioning Certificate
Frank Powell, Deacon

Special    "So Send I You"    Mim Hostetler

Hymn 372

Benediction

Refreshments follow in the all-purpose room
Everyone welcome

## COMMISSIONING THOUGHTS

Our Lord gave his disciples this commission: "Go, therefore, and make disciples of all nations". Missions is so fundamental throughout the Scriptures and found to be the purpose of the Church.

But, "thanks be to God" there is not the "go" without the, "Lo, I am with you always!". It is God that worketh in you both to do and to will according to his good pleasure. When I was a child and several times since, God has confirmed His will for my life and it is upon that knowledge and with that security I can now step forward as a medical missionary.

Now is the beginning of a very new year and a good time for each of us to make goals and changes; to sit back to see where one's life has been and the direction in which it is going. I trust you will be willing to give your best of anything to Him. It is then that we are the clay and He, the Potter. We can have the kind of faith it takes to be molded because He is trustworthy.

While the service tonight is not a farewell, I would like to just take this opportunity to say I love you, each one, and will be praying for you, too, in the time we are apart. Please forgive me for the tears and, if I do not see each of you before I leave, then it's OK because that is pretty hard for me. I will remember you, each one.

One last comment I would make of sentimental value is that the brooch/locket I am wearing tonight was given to Agnes Hathaway, a missionary in Japan and the daughter of my Great-grandfather Jones, cousin. It is a Hartwig family keepsake.

I have so many fond memories of this church family that will also be "keepsakes" and sustaining.

In God's service,
Barb

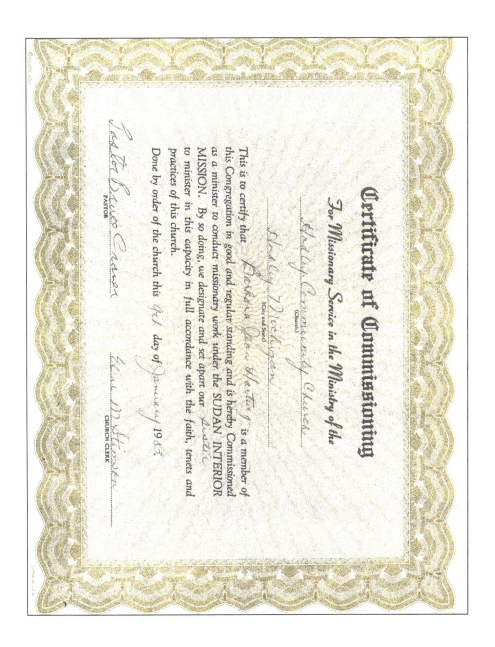

# PART TWO

## ASSIGNMENT: LIBERIA

### 1983-1992

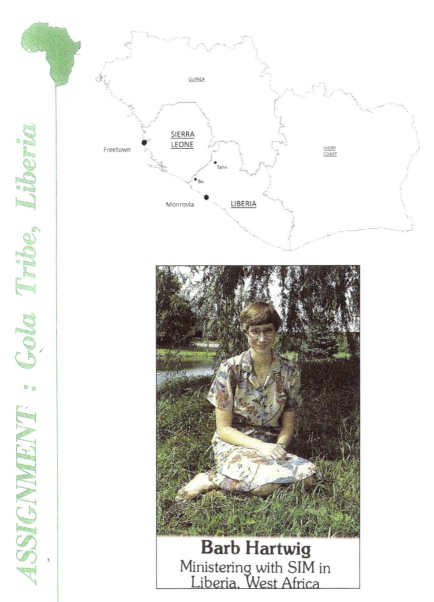

## CHAPTER 5

ASSIGNMENT : Gola Tribe, Liberia

GUINEA

SIERRA
LEONE

Freetown

IVORY
COAST

Tahn

Bo

Monrovia    LIBERIA

**Barb Hartwig**
Ministering with SIM in
Liberia, West Africa

# ASSIGNMENT: GOLA TRIBE, LIBERIA (1983–1989)

*I finally arrived* on the mission field February 18, 1983! I was twenty-seven years old.

Jessica Layman and I traveled together from the JFK Airport in New York City, across the Atlantic Ocean via Brussels, to Monrovia, Liberia. The heat and humidity hit me as I stepped off the big plane, but I remember smiling and being happy to be there. The difficult farewells and preparations were all behind!

SIM's Liberia headquarters is on the 137 acre Atlantic coastal property deeded to the mission in 1952. It is just south of the capital city, Monrovia. The international Christian radio station with the call letters ELWA, standing for Eternal Love Winning Africa, is also the name of SIM's big mission station. ELWA Radio aired broadcasts in forty different languages. ELWA was quite popular and had an incredibly good reputation. Radio was popular because of the high rate of illiteracy and remoteness of so many Liberians. Broadcasters in local languages would give announcements as sent in to them. Not only was ELWA Radio on the coastal property, but eventually there was ELWA Hospital, ELWA Academy, a print shop, guest house, carpenter shop, services, and an International Church. The Mission administration offices and treasury were in the radio studio building, which had a huge antenna field around it. All of these ministries were packed in between the beautiful Atlantic beach lined with coconut trees and houses, and the public road. We had three-quarters of a mile of coastline, some of which was great for swimming. No one imagined the magnet this compound would become during the civil war to both displaced people and warlords.

Jessica and I were "adopted" by ELWA missionaries Brian and Ruth Clark from the time we arrived. Our friendship has been a rock and mutual help to each other through some future difficult times, right up to today. Brian was field treasurer and Ruth worked in the clinic. When Liberia "crashed" in 1990, the Clarks were reassigned to Ethiopia, and I went there, too, in 1993 (see the Ethiopia chapter to read about Ruth's tragic car accident that left her paralyzed in Ethiopia in 1996). Ruth has been my dear friend and counselor; my go-to person innumerable times for Godly wisdom and advice.

Jessica and I were invited to many different missionaries' homes for a meal during our first week in Liberia. Hospitality is a wonderful ministry in Africa. All my experience with cooking and baking while growing up would come into good use overseas, as I often had guests and friends over for a meal. I helped Jessica get settled into her new apartment just a few miles from ELWA. She joined some other single ladies who were also teaching Religious Knowledge classes in public schools across Monrovia. After a lot of orientation, meetings, shopping for groceries downtown, money exchange, etc., I was anxious to see my new home at Tahn! Jessica accompanied me there.

On Saturday February 26, Dr. Steve Befus, Jessica, two medical students named Sarah and Marilee, and I drove two hours to Tahn with our pickup loaded to the hilt with seven of my boxes and Renate's new desk. We arrived just in time for the Village Health Workers meeting Steve had arranged. Steve led the meeting with seventeen or so village health workers (VHW) who attended from all over the Gola District. Joy Crombie had trained them, but she was still at home in New Zealand on extended furlough. Steve introduced me as the new nurse joining Miss Crombie! What an honor and overwhelming responsibility on my first day at Tahn. By the grace of God I felt up to this challenge with zeal and great interest in all that the team at Tahn was doing. Finally, in the afternoon, we ate our packed lunch. I remember that the station "pet" mongoose named Arnold had gotten into the truck and had eaten Sarah's lunch. Renate Isert and Libby Kindall were the single gals at Tahn, and we all shared our food after the meeting. Dr. Steve, Jessica, Sarah and Marilee drove back to ELWA later that afternoon. I unpacked a bit at the house I was to share with Renate until our duplex was built. Renate and I sat on our screened-in verandah that evening and spent the time getting acquainted. It was wonderful to be a part of this church-planting team!

Two couples important to the mission at Tahn were still back at ELWA in Monrovia the day I arrived. Les and Verla Unruh started church planting in the Gola District in 1979 and were our leaders at Tahn when

I arrived. This was the first church-planting outreach SIM did in Liberia. The Unruhs built a small mission compound just north of Tahn Village. There were four houses and seven missionaries at Tahn in 1983. Ben and Monie Motis were teaching at the Bible School for church leaders. Monie was a literacy teacher. Life was comfortable. We had pre-fab steel housing units; running water pumped from a well; a generator for some evening power; bottle gas stoves and little refrigerators. The Tahn church-planting team had a good reputation as a team of individuals, for each member brought specific skills and were committed to working hard toward the goal of seeing the church established and nurtured.

My specific assignment included Gola language study for three months with Renate Isert's supervision. I did that, but it was not a full-time assignment. The Community Based Health Care (CBHC) program, started by Joy Crombie, interested me considerably. Les and Verla gave me the key to Joy's house and said to just go in and read all her records to learn what the program was about. Looking through her office cupboards, it looked like she had trained a lot of health workers and traditional midwives! She kept good notes and I figured out a lot of what she had done. She also had many books and articles about community health, which I spent hours devouring.

Before I finished my three-month Gola language study, another opportunity for ministry popped up. The Tahn School principal came to Les one day and asked him for a missionary to teach Religious Knowledge (RK) classes at the local school. The principal said if we didn't send someone, he would have to let the Muslim Imam in to teach. Les asked me to do it, and I agreed. So in April (their school year starts in April) I started teaching Bible classes three mornings a week to the sixth-, seventh-, and eighth-graders, one hour a week with each class. Each week I typed up their lesson on a stencil and hand cranked the stencil machine to run off copies. I ended up doing this the whole seven and a half years I lived at Tahn. God gave me this opportunity to get involved in peoples' lives. The students often came to visit me on my veranda to ask questions, do homework, or read the many books I left out on the porch table for them. I loved this opportunity and was soon more involved in my local community through the school and students! The RK class's impact on students' lives cannot be measured in numbers, but I know God spoke to these kids as I opened up the Word of God to them.

One day I was studying Gola when Abraham Ware, the Tahn government clinic worker, came to my house to report a measles outbreak at one village. He said we needed to take measles vaccine to them as soon as possible. Okay, yes, but I did not know how to do this. I read up on measles and vaccines at Joy's house. Les and Verla ordered the vaccine from ELWA Hospital, and it came up in a cold box with someone traveling to Tahn. ELWA radio broadcasted the announcement of our upcoming vaccination clinic. The day came and Abraham and I went to the village. It was my first community health outreach, and I was hooked. The community-based type of health work was going to suit me just fine. I never did work in a hospital or clinic in Africa during my whole twenty-eight years there. And that was not for want of being asked to do curative work many times! My reasons are forthcoming in chapter 13.

Another opportunity for Bible teaching came my way when Verla Unruh handed over her girls' Sunday School class to me at the Tahn church. God answered prayers as I sought out appropriate lessons to teach them and developed rapport with the girls. One of the girls was named Elizabeth. Her parents were Muslim and her father was the town chief. Elizabeth and her sister Maria finished eighth grade at Tahn school and wanted to attend high school. The nearest high school was an hour away at Bomi Hills. Long story short, Beth and Maria did go to high school at Bomi Hills, and Jessica and I paid their room rent. If I remember right, they were the first girls from Tahn to graduate from high school! Beth remained faithful to God throughout those years and met her future husband, Tony Weedor, during that time. Beth has written a book of her life history called *Out of the Ashes,* by Elizabeth Fahn Weedor. I highly recommend this account of her early life at Tahn, her high school years at Bomi Hills, her marriage to Tony, and their survival during the civil war in Liberia.

I hit the ground running at Tahn. What with Gola language study, Religious Knowledge classes at school in town, village health outreach, the girls' Sunday School class, a mid-week Children's Bible Club at Harrisfield village, missionary health care and hospitality, life was very, very busy. I thrived on all of it.

One important place on our mission compound was the *palaver* hut. *Palaver* means "discussion or even argument" in Liberian English. It was grass roofed with a round sitting area, and had a cement floor and a short wall around it in between the doorway spaces. It had a good breeze and view of the station! Lots of meetings and visits from people were held at the *palaver* hut. Speaking of Liberian English, I was immersed in it. I learned to both understand and speak it. I can still speak it today. Doing so was essential to the ministry work, as it is the trade language of Liberia. One might have to humble oneself to speak it, but the smiles it will bring from the Liberians are all it takes to learn it. I never was fluent in the Gola language, but I could speak Liberian English and use a Gola interpreter when necessary. My theory is that language learning is a gift somewhat related to music, of which I never did have the wherewithal to excel in. I believe that people who can carry a tune are more inclined to do well picking up another language—just my opinion.

Later in 1983 Ron Sonius, Les Unruh, and Ben Motis finished building a duplex on the station out of donated prefab materials. Renate and I moved in, and I was so happy to have my own place at Tahn. As already mentioned, my screened-in veranda was very popular because kids from town/school/church would come and sit and read or ask questions. Sometimes they had to entertain themselves. I had a local hammock on my veranda, which made for a great siesta spot, too! There was some breeze out there, whereas inside the house was stifling hot during the day. How hot? I don't know because I made it my policy in Africa not to know the actual temperature in and outside. I truly believe that knowing how hot it is in the dry season makes one feel worse. Here is the general dry season (November to April) weather report for sub-Sahara Africa: Hot with a chance of hotter!

Ben and Monie Motis and their two kids, Tim and Cathy, took over as district superintendent for SIM after the Unruhs left Liberia to work in SIM's home office in Charlotte, North Carolina. They were also absolutely wonderful to work with. Once in a while Monie would go out and turn on the generator for a few minutes on a very hot afternoon to blend Orange Julius or banana shakes for everyone! Ben was always there if we had a problem, but otherwise he just let us loose to expand the community health program. Marianne Atzbach from Germany arrived in 1984. She was a nurse and joined Joy and me in the program until Joy was transferred to start up a new health program in Liberia's Kolahun District. Ray and Jayne Hutchison and their two little boys arrived to take over the Gola Bible School training when Ben stepped up to be District

Superintendent. I always admired Ray and Jayne for their gift of evangelism and outreach to the Liberians.

One of the special things we did as a team was celebrate Ben and Monie's twenty-fifth anniversary at Tahn. We organized a progressive dinner for them one evening. They started out at one of our houses for salad with candlelight and music by themselves, and we even gave them some possible topics for conversation. Then they went to another house for the main meal, including Ray's famous french fries, and then to another house for dessert. We gave it our best shot to make it a memorable evening for them. On the mission field, the smaller things and homemade things meant a whole lot more. Too often our busy schedules and jobs cause us to miss opportunities to "do unto others. . ." We were a pretty good church-planting team at Tahn. Looking out for others is partly why.

Suddenly, on June 4, 1984, I received news from home that my dad had had a heart attack! He was only fifty-five years old. I remember taking public transport in a taxi to Monrovia so I could phone home. Then on October 28, 1984, I received word that Dad had suffered a cardiac arrest and almost didn't make it to the hospital. Wow. I went home. He had triple bypass surgery in November, and I took early furlough until March of 1985. He recovered and by the grace of God lived another eleven years. One fun thing I got to do on this unexpected short winter furlough, was be a bridesmaid in Jessica's wedding . Jessica met Steve Longabaugh in Monrovia. They fell in love, got married and after Steve joined SIM, they joined the SIM team in Guinea ( a neighboring country to Liberia).

In 1985, when I returned from my short furlough, I spent two weeks at ELWA Hospital training with the Liberian midwives. I needed hands-on experience working with labor and delivery patients. It was very helpful. Then I attended a WHO/UNICEF training-of-trainers course on how to work with traditional birth attendants (TBA) and train them. These are the grandmothers who do most of the baby deliveries in rural Africa. I learned how to work with illiterate women and teach them clean delivery techniques; as well as how to recognize complications and refer women to the hospital hopefully in time to save the baby and mother. Joy Crombie taught me a lot, but this official training grounded me with broad knowledge and some skills in midwifery. We were supervising forty-two trained traditional midwives by the time the civil war started. I took this training in Liberia with me to Ghana and South Sudan, where I also trained and supervised TBAs.

December, 1986, and January, 1987, are memorable for several reasons. Ray and Jayne Hutchison came down with Hepatitis at the same time! They had four children by then, including sixteen-month-old twins. As mentioned, Ray and Jayne had taken over the Gola Bible School from Ben and Monie so Ben could focus on church planting. Only the Motises, Marianna, and I were on the station to take turns caring for the kids when they got sick. Ray found it very hard to stay in bed. The only treatment for Hepatitis is rest and plenty of good food. So I would tell Ray to go back to bed and get well! That is how he could help. But to this day, he calls me "Sarge" because of that! All in good humor to be sure. One evening, Marianne was "on duty" at their house, but she soon came to me and asked, "How do you make grilled cheese sandwiches?" That is what sounded good to Ray and Jayne. Apparently, they do not make this type of sandwich in Germany. I explained how to do it, but Marianne just turned around and went home. I went and prepared dinner up there.

Oh, I was hoping I did not contract hepatitis too, because my mother and her sister, Aunt Lucy Brushaber, were due to arrive in January for a two-week visit! How exciting and how I looked forward to this! I had everything planned. Well, they came, and I didn't get sick.

How wonderful to introduce my mother and aunt to all the people I worked with! It was the only time I had family visit except when my niece Rachel came to Ghana with our Hadley church youth group in 2004 when she was only thirteen years old. It was so much fun to show Mom and Aunt Lucy around ELWA, Tahn, and several of the villages we worked in. My parents and siblings were staunch supporters of my missionary work the whole thirty years. They recognized God's call on my life. I do not take that lightly, because I know many fellow missionaries over the years who did not have that kind of family support, and it was hard for them to stay. I praise the Lord for my family, who did not pressure me to come home, even after the close calls that happened. My mother was a great partner with me in this cross-culture work. She wrote me letters, sent packages, mailed out all my prayer letters to about five hundred addresses three or four times a year, prayed for me, and did so many errands for me stateside. Those were the days before computer and phones made instant communications possible, so we relied on mail a lot.

Marianne and I partnered in the Community Based Health Care work. We trained and supervised sixteen village health workers (VHW) and forty-two trained traditional birth attendants (TBA) from about nineteen villages. Every Friday we did an immunization clinic at one of those villages. That was a lot of work. Ordering and reporting on vaccines from UNICEF in Monrovia was no small task. Sometimes, we had huge turnouts on Fridays because we informed the village leaders ahead of time of our arrival by letter and ELWA broadcasts. A typical Friday went like this. We packed up our pickup early with plenty of supplies that we had prepped the day before. Arriving at the village, we greeted the chief, church leaders, VHWs, and TBAs. We usually set up our work area in a *palaver* hut in the village. When a crowd gathered, either Marianna or I gave devotions and prayed. One of us filled out the "Road To Health" cards recording the vaccines needing to be given that day, weighed the child and put that on his growth chart to see if he was growing, and then explained all to his or her mother. The other one of us gave the vaccines, which were dated to be given that day. Marianne and I took turns in those two roles. Most kids resisted us and it was difficult to give the vaccines. By the time we finished in the afternoon, we were totally exhausted. Yet we still had pregnant women to check with the TBAs and sick kids to treat. We also restocked our volunteer VHW's medicine supplies. By the time we drove back to Tahn late in the afternoon, neither of us had an energy left. Almost every Friday we did these outreach clinics.

Over the years I received innumerable requests to visit a sick family member and administer some kind of help, which I willingly did. Many times I did what I could and also referred them to the local government clinic. Abraham Ware was a good physician assistant, but he was gone a lot. I recall a young woman in the Tahn Church who had seizures. She needed help and I knew what to do. James 4:17 says, "Therefore, to one who knows the right thing to do, and does not do it, to him it is sin." I was convicted, and so I took her to ELWA clinic in Monrovia to be diagnosed and started on medicine. The first medicine they prescribed for epilepsy caused severe side effects for her. They changed it to phenobarbital, and once regulated, it controlled her seizures and changed her life completely. This is just one example of the pressure on me to do curative medicine. I was not trained in diagnosis and treatment. And I never wanted to do that level of health work. But over the years, I had to use my medical textbooks and prescribe medicine the best I could in many situations with God's help and a prayer. How many people were drawn into the church because someone visited them while sick and prayed for them and helped them get better? Tons. Sometimes, I wrote on a piece of paper what they should go to the local "pharmacy" and buy. Even that seemingly insignificant help was enough and so appreciated.

My first seven-plus years in Africa were good years. I loved my work and the people around me, both the Liberian nationals and missionaries. Having this good start would serve me well in some tough times ahead. The 1980s were years that grounded me in a lot of African culture.

Let me summarize our Gola church-planting strategy and work in these years before the civil war. To my best recollection, we had eight churches established in the Gola District. A church was basically defined as having at least ten members and two church leaders. Preaching points were places that did not meet that definition yet, but often an evangelist would go there to preach. Les, Ben, and Ray worked diligently to develop leadership. We had meetings with leaders. We had the Bible School. Ben did some TEE classes (Theological Education by Extension), but attendance was always up and down. Sometimes, Ben would go off on his motorcycle for a meeting, and no one would show up. Our annual Gola Church conference every January was the highlight of the year! It was a very special gathering of all churches, preaching points, missionaries, and many from the town hosting the conference that year.

I quote from my March, 1989, prayer letter: "On the last night of Conference, I had one of those precious moments in life that makes everything sacrificed worthwhile. We had been showing one of the four-part series of "Jesus" films each night after the preaching. The last film depicts Christ being crucified and then resurrected. It is very moving and realistic. Many adults came for counseling afterwards. When almost everyone was gone, I was helping take down the white sheet used for a screen when I turned and saw a boy from Harrisfield kneeling and praying at the front of the church. I knew him well from my weekly Bible class there. Sitting beside him, I asked, "Shall I pray for you?" I did, and then said, "Now you pray," which he did in his own dialect. Only God knows what he prayed, but I felt somehow that here was someone

39

spiritually born-again with repentance and acceptance in his heart. What a great way to begin this new term here among the Gola people."

I close this chapter with some explanation of what we were up against as a church. The two religions in the area were Folk Islam and animism, or Traditional African Religion (TAR). Folk Islam is a mixture of traditional religion and Islam. Animism is an indigenous religion attributing spirits to inanimate objects. One might then worship a created thing, such as a tree or a rock. Ancestor worship is part of TAR. A witch doctor or soothsayer would advise someone what to do for a problem. And not for free, either. For example, if one wanted protection from sickness for their child, the witch doctor would tell them what amulet or fetish to put on the child and charge them money for it. It was very, very difficult for a Christian to completely leave the TAR beliefs he or she grew up with. So one might keep, or syncretize, some of them with either Folk Islam or Christianity. One cannot but admit the existence of supernatural forces associated with animism too. Fear of men and evil spirits characterizes the animist believer. A Christian coming out of this background needs discipling to read God's Word; he needs kindness and love and security; he needs to be able to go to the pastor for advice instead of the witch doctor; he needs someone to show him from Scripture, for example, what Gideon did with his father's idols.

In 1984 a crises developed. The lead Gola Pastor was Varney and his wife Mary. Their twelve year old daughter, Neor, was kidnapped by the TAR Sande (women's) Bush Society. Neor was taken without parental permission for the purpose of initiation into the Society by means of female circumcision. The parents went to the police and district officials but were told it was a matter for the traditional governing authorities (chiefs). Pastor Varney appealed to the chiefs, but to no avail. Pastor and Mary eventually knew where she was being held, but she would not or could not come out. She was initiated as far as I know.

In my first week in Liberia in February 1983, one of the first culture lessons Jessica and I learned was not to interfere in the Bush Society, and that only the national church leaders knew how to address this powerful entity. So we stood by and prayed when Neor was taken.

Space will not permit me to explain all the ways animism was intertwined in Liberians' lives. One principle that I think the church should abide by, though, is that if you take something away, then fill the gap with something else. For example, if the church says do not go to the witch doctor, then people should go to the pastor for advice and Biblical counseling. If the church says do not initiate with circumcision, then it needs to replace that rite of passage with something else.

I found that the four main barriers to being a Christian or being a committed Christian were: illiteracy, Islam/animism, immorality, and idleness.

One of the first things you will find as a barrier to friendship with women in rural Africa is that most do not speak English and cannot read. Their children and their farm are their lives. Girls that go to school are likely to have self-esteem and confidence, and can rise above superstitions, adapt to changes from tradition, listen to healthier ways to live, and can read the Bible. Barriers for girls to stay in school are if it is not safe for them to walk to school, they have poor teachers, or there is not enough money for uniforms and shoes for sons and daughters. Rules such as she must stay home when she has her period, or if she gets pregnant, make it very difficult to attend when the teenage years come. Parents will usually not send all their children to school. Some must stay home and work on the farm. The odds of Marie and Elizabeth, who I mentioned earlier in this chapter, graduating from high school in Liberia were so low, but God came into their lives and nothing is impossible with Him!

I close this chapter with a few bits and pieces of life in Liberia:

It's 110 degrees in the shade!
The farmer's main farming tool called a cutlass is made by a blacksmith from car springs.
Rubber "shoes" made from tires are sold in the local market.
"The twins were born 4 months apart."
Billy selling thorn carvings at ELWA beach.
We are from the same ma, same pa!
Red clay dirt up country.
White egrets, the Christmas birds, seen mixing with the cows in December.
Open markets come to town every six days.
Sudden service (fast food) advertised at King Burger in Monrovia
BBC radio news on shortwave stations.
Checkpoints along the roads.
Kwii, meaning western.

No running hot water for dishes or bathing.

A sassa and drums to accompany singing at church.

Frangipani trees, bougainvillea, hibiscus, poinsettia trees, coconut, and palm nut trees.

Vacations with Laura Miller at Voice of America compound and Africa Bible College campus.

My cousin Wayne writing "keep your chin up and your head down" after the close call.

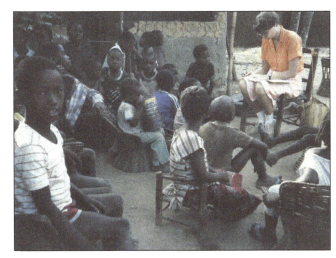

Teaching kids at a weekly Bible club at Harrisfield village.

I taught "Religious Knowledge" classes at Tahn School for seven years.

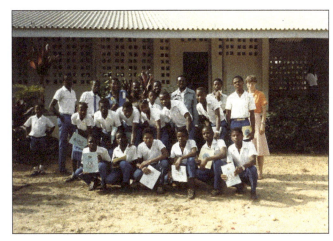

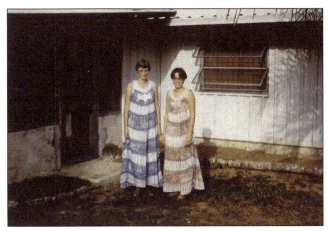

Jessica Layman and I dressed up for annual Gola church conference: this picture was taken in front of my prefab. house at Tahn

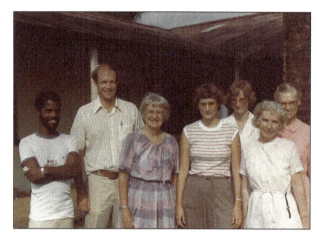

Community Health Worker Team:
Abraham Ware (Tahn clinic)
Dr. Steve Befus
Joy Crombie
Me
(Not sure who is in the white uniform)
Marianne Atzbach
Libby Muchmore

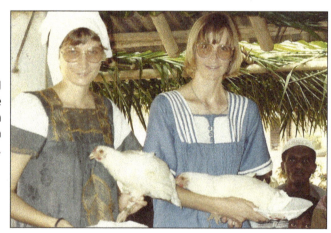

Marianne and I accept live gifts at a graduation ceremony.

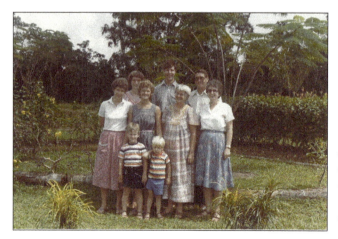

Our Tahn missionary team:
Back:
Marianne Atzbach
Ray Hutchison
Ben Motis

Front: Renate Isert
Jayne Hutchison
Joy Crombie
Monie Motis
Boys Josh and Joel Hutchison

.LAPEER, MICHIGAN       *4 MARCH 1987*

## A visit to West Africa

# HADLEY NEWS

*by BARB ZALEWSKI*

Bev Hartwig just returned from a two week visit with her missionary daughter, Barb, over in Liberia, West Africa, in a little village called Tahn where Barb lives and works.

Bev and her sister Lucy, from Florida, flew over to see the type of work Barb does. They met the peole who make up her 'other family' as well as enjoyed some time together.

She learned how the Nationals (the people wish to be called Nationals, not natives) are learning health care and the necessity of cleanliness, as well as the control on communicable diseases by vaccination.

Barb is a nurse and has Bible College training, which enables her to teach Bible stories and songs to the women and children. The mortality rate for newborns has dropped considerably since the training of midwives began.

Bev said the people were shy at first, but were soon talking and sharing. They are very strong on 'family' and it's obvious. They love their children very much.

It was a great experience for Bev and Lucy to get to make this trip. They even had a shopping trip in Amsterdam on the way home. It's something you dream about, but never expect it to really happen! But — dreams do come true, don't they Bev?

Article in The County Press

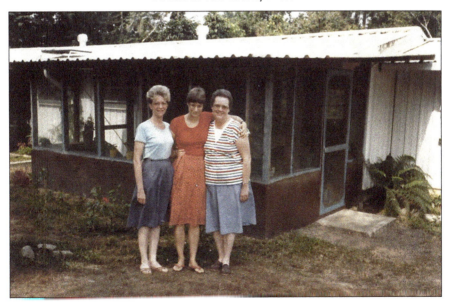

Aunt Lucy Brushaber, me, and my mother Beverly,
standing in front of my house at Tahn when they visited
Liberia in 1987.

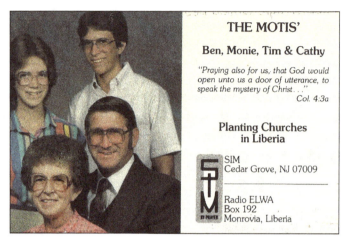

THE MOTIS'

Ben, Monie, Tim & Cathy

*"Praying also for us, that God would open unto us a door of utterance, to speak the mystery of Christ..."*
Col. 4:3a

**Planting Churches in Liberia**

SIM
Cedar Grove, NJ 07009

Radio ELWA
Box 192
Monrovia, Liberia

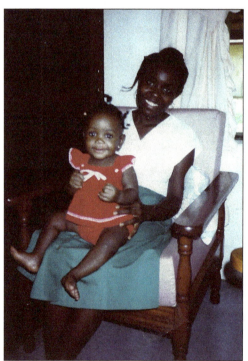

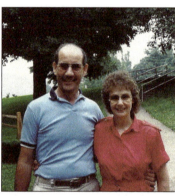

Les and Verla Unruh, who started the church-planting work in Liberia at Tahn.

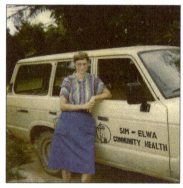

Meet Elizabeth Fahn-Weedor and her daughter. She and her sister Marie are from Tahn and graduated from high school, the first girls from that village to do so.

CHAPTER 6

# DETAINED AT THE BORDER (1990).
# CLOSE CALL #1

*The civil war* in Liberia started on Christmas Eve, December 24, 1989. It ended fourteen years later. The country imploded, self-destructed, and had no central government until the election in 1997. Trusting God, no matter what, came to the test when we were detained at the border in July of 1990.

Most of our ELWA missionaries evacuated Monrovia in April, 1990. A handful of men and women remained at ELWA in Monrovia until the same day Ben and Monie Motis, their kids, Tim and Cathy, and I left on July 28, 1990. The ELWA group left via the Ivory Coast border, and we left via the Sierra Leone border. Those months between April and July are a long and complicated story.

To learn what happened simultaneously to our departure to Sierra Leone, I refer to Bill Ardill's book *Where Elephants Fight* for an autobiographical account of their time at ELWA station in Monrovia.

In May there were five missionaries left at Tahn, plus the Motises' two college-age kids, Tim and Cathy, who were "home" for the summer visiting Ben and Monie. On May 28 we received word via radio from our field Director Jon Shea that a strong rumor said there was a Charles Taylor rebel group coming to our Cape Mount County. Jon said we had to leave Tahn immediately. We opted to drive to the Kolahun area and join our fellow SIM missionaries there instead of leaving Liberia. Little did we know it was a very rough road, or lack thereof, over a mountain, to get from Tahn to Kolahun. Our caravan got stuck and spent a long night on that mountain in our vehicles. We left Renate's Suzuki there with a burned-out clutch. When the seven of us arrived at Kolahun, a district meeting was held with us. Renate and Marianne decided to leave Liberia via Guinea with some Southern Baptist missionaries named Ken and Joyce Nicholson.

I had a big decision to make. I could either leave with Marianne and Renate, and Ken and Joyce, or stay on with Ben and Monie. Interestingly, my father got in touch with Jon Shea at ELWA while we were en route to Kolahun and asked if I was coming home. Jon answered my dad for me and said I would be staying with the Motises. Apparently, my dad did not ask me to come home. If my father or field director had told me to leave, I would have. I wished I could have talked with my dad myself and was surprised that Jon Shea had answered for me. One reason I did not leave via Guinea with Renate and Marianne was because I did not have a credit card or access to enough money to buy a ticket home out of Guinea. I decided to stay and leave when and if Ben and Monie did. I believe God led me so, because later on, when Ben was so sick with severe malaria, I had the quinine medicine he needed to recover. (I have diary notes of all I did between May and July up in the Kolahun area, but have decided not to put it in this account.)

In early July, we knew the rebels were coming to the Kolahun area. Soon after, Ben and Monie and I decided to leave Liberia, but via Tahn. The missionaries in Kolahun District who did stay for the rebel take-over there were not treated well and received serious threats against them. To avoid the mountain that gave us so much trouble on the way over, we went via a road that touched into Sierra Leone, picking up passengers along the way to guide us. We started to encounter some anti-America sentiment at checkpoints. It was a two-day trip back to Tahn. Cape Mount County was the last county in Liberia uninvaded by the rebels, but we were still leaving. We arrived back on a Wednesday, and Ben said we'll leave Saturday morning and go to Sierra Leone to wait there and see what happens in Liberia. In Sierra Leone, Tim and Cathy could get back to college with their round-trip tickets out of Freetown. I carefully packed one big suitcase at Tahn. We arranged for guards at our neat little compound home just outside of the village of Tahn. We talked with church leaders and community workers/leaders. The day before we left Tahn, I baked a double or triple batch of chocolate chip cookies for our trip. Our "neighbors" with the Wesleyan Mission, with whom we could communicate via radio, left the area the day before we were leaving and had no trouble. Our local authorities required us to travel with a soldier for protection and to clear our way through checkpoints.

Paul and Laura (pseudo names) were acquaintances of ours in the Tahn area. They came to Ben and asked to go "out" with us. They were Christians. Paul had a diamond washing "operation" of some sort along Lofa River, and Laura worked as a librarian in Monrovia most of the time. Ben agreed to give them a ride to Sierra Leone. Now we were seven Americans leaving in three vehicles.

On that Saturday morning, we left Tahn early and arrived at the border station called Bo to leave Liberia. This is at the big Mano River bridge (see the postcard picture of it at the end of this chapter). Sierra Leone was on the other side of this bridge. We had to see the immigration office people in order to leave. Liberia police and soldiers were swarming all over the place. For two hours there was no trouble, and we were finally ready to leave in our three vehicles. Suddenly one soldier came around, looked at me in the driver's seat of the Land Cruiser, and said to me, "You're going back to Monrovia." It was our first inkling of trouble. Soon more soldiers gathered around our vehicles. The immigration man came out and said, "Give me all your passports." We gave them back and never saw them again. He said, "We have just received a radio message from the Mansion that there are nine missionaries coming to cross the border today, and we are to send them back to Monrovia. So park your vehicles over there." We did. Ben and Paul tried to talk to them, but to no avail. We heard another one of the men say, "America is aiding the rebels." The government soldiers and police were upset with America. America did have a ship sitting offshore of Monrovia, standing by for our American embassy people in case they needed to evacuate. America had not, however, taken a side in the conflict between President Samuel Doe and Rebel leader Charles Taylor.

The immigration man started to call us into his office one at a time for questioning. Tim went first and was in his office for at least an hour. Then he called in Monie. When he called me in, he asked, "Why didn't you go home when your embassy told you to?" "Where are you coming from?" "What work do you do?" "Why were you at Upper Lofa?" Rather abruptly he stopped interrogating me and said he was tired and sick and going home. He ordered me to go back to the car. It was 6 p.m. Ben asked him what we should do, and he said he did not know. Clearly we would not be allowed to leave Liberia.

Paul's Liberian partner, Seku, was with us too. He was free to go anywhere he wanted. Ben and Paul got a piece of paper and wrote down our seven names, gave Seku some money, and asked him to take our note to the American embassy in Freetown, Sierra Leone. He agreed and left us. For a week, we never knew if he made it to the Embassy or not, but he had. I actually saw the very slip of paper with our names on it in the file of the political officer who debriefed us a week later. And that is how the American government and SIM knew we were in trouble at the border.

We remained in our three vehicles all Saturday night. A generator had come on and one big flood light. We parked right in the middle of that light and were dozing. The battery in my watch had died sometime in April so I never knew the exact time. It was around 3 a.m. when we all woke up suddenly and saw people running around everywhere. Crowds of people were moving towards the bridge and leaving Liberia. We could hear hollering coming from a prisoner in jail just behind us. He was eerily yelling, "Let me out of here." Soon one man came running nearby, and seeing our confusion, he said to us, "The rebels are coming." Feeling the impending danger, we huddled and decided to try to leave, too. We started up our vehicles, Ben driving the truck in front. I was driving a Land Cruiser. We got up to the gate and a couple guys said, "Aww, let them go," but others with guns pointed at Ben and said, "Uh-uh. You're not going anywhere." Ben started to argue and they said, "Get back or we'll shoot." I started backing up immediately and Ben did, too. We saw an empty room and parked near it. So we took our belongings out of the vehicles and went in.

Paul convinced us to try giving them money. Ben was definitely not in favor of this, but Paul said he would handle it. He took $500 USD and went to try to find out who was in charge. He found one named Colonel Lincoln and another guy who seemed a bit sympathetic to our situation. Paul was making a deal to get our passports back and permission to cross the bridge. They demanded $100 per passport. So Paul gave them $700. Lincoln said we had to go right then and that he would bring us the passports. It was early morning as we drove up to the gate again, and after much discussion, they lifted the gate bar and we drove on. I was in the lead vehicle this time. We got halfway across the bridge, when one lone soldier with a gun stepped out from behind a parked van and pointed his long gun right at me, saying, "Get back. Get back." His finger was on the trigger. I started to back up. No discussion necessary. We went back to the empty building and never saw Lincoln again.

The second man who was with Lincoln when Paul paid them was there at the immigration building and said to me, "Back it up." Then he said, "Put your load down," then, "Put that seat up," followed by "Give me the key." He took off.

They confiscated both of our Land Cruisers, which left us very shaken and scared. Someone came and told us to move out, because they were using the room. We were at a loss, standing around outside, but then someone came and told us to go into the customs room down at the end of the building. Most of the front of the room was open. We decided to build ourselves a barricade at the back of the customs room with two huge old desks, an old freezer, and an engine block. At least we had a place to hide, out of sight, when the rebels arrived. In one more attempt, Ben and Paul actually tried to walk up to the gate again, but they were turned back at gunpoint.

It had been raining all night and morning. A soldier was sitting outside our room, in front of the building. He was guarding us, but we were free to wander around. We had little to no desire to do so with all the anti-America sentiment around there.

The soldier who had pointed the gun at Ben the first time we tried to leave was very angry and came to lecture us about how bad America was for not helping the government. His conclusion was, "You are here until the war is over." We did not try to talk to him, only listened. We finally accepted the fact that we were there for the coming battle. It was Sunday. Nobody wanted to eat. We spent most of our time near the barricade. We thought we would most likely get caught in the middle of their fight.

We waited . . . and waited all day. Some Gola people we knew who were part of the crowd rushing to leave came to sympathize with us, although they were leery of being seen as friendly. When Matthew and Victor from Harrisfield (the village where I had taught the kids weekly Bible Club) left, they said they would get their families across and come back and negotiate for us. I had tears in my eyes when I heard him say that. I appreciated it so much.

A couple of guys who happened to be Korean came in with their truck. Ben had a chance to quickly tell them what was going on and asked them to report our situation to the American embassy in Freetown. They nodded and said they would.

It was now about 5 p.m. and I had just gone out and brushed my teeth. I came back and found Ben secretly listening to the BBC on radio. I sat on the desk and was thinking about eating something. By now we thought we were here for the night. The rebels would not come today, and we were all dreading the night and figuring they would likely attack at daybreak. Suddenly, shooting started up all over the place. I jumped off the desk and dived over the barricade. I happened to land between Monie and Cathy, who were already on the floor. Laura and Paul were also already behind the barricade. So was Tim because he had a bad headache. I was almost caught outside when the fighting started. Or did the rebels wait until I got back inside? I figure the rebels were hiding around the place and saw me go out and return! Ben dived in right in front of Cathy.

The shooting was intense. At one point, Paul shouted, "We need a white flag." Laura said, "I have a white slip." Paul told her to take it off. There was glass breaking, something hitting the roof, and it was all very loud. People were screaming. Monie and I were gripping hands. Ben and Cathy were gripping hands. Ben said we lay there a whole hour. Later Monie told us that she was praying for God to take us all if we must die. I hoped she did not mean me too, but whoever her prayer included, God spared our lives. By a miracle, not a single bullet that we know of entered the inside of that room that had no front wall. At the first lull, Ben spoke and Paul raised the white flag because we had to identify ourselves to the rebels. We didn't know if any soldiers were also hiding in the room. After a peek, Ben and Paul saw rebels out there

Ben hollered out, "Missionaries! American missionaries!" The rebel guy heard him and saw our flag, and ordered us all to come out! He asked us if we had any soldiers with us. We said no, and that we were ELWA missionaries and the soldiers would not let us cross the border. They asked if this was our truck.

Then they said to us, "We are Freedom Fighters. We come here. We protect you, we protect you. You free now, feel free, you are all right now."

We could still hear some shooting outside. He saw that we ladies were still afraid and he didn't like that. He told us nothing could happen to us now. Finally, Monie, Cathy, Laura, and I got into the back of our pickup truck. I tried not to be afraid because the freedom fighter really did not like us looking afraid. I guess he thought we did not trust them to protect us if we were still afraid.

Then the freedom fighter helped Ben and the guys put our things into the truck. We just wanted to leave, stuff or not. That's when our helper saw our cookies. He asked for one and Ben said, "Yes, you can have them all." He shared them around in good Liberian style. There were only about twenty Freedom Fighters, and they were very hungry. The fighter who picked up my rice bag to load it must have seen my Liberian money and took it. Later when I realized it, we did not say anything. It wasn't worth getting him beat or even killed because he probably was not supposed to do that.

The Freedom Fighters said we could leave. We barely started to drive up to the bridge gateway when some of the Freedom Fighters said they saw some government soldiers escape that way and were not sure if they might be hiding on or near the bridge. They said it would be dangerous to cross. So the Freedom Fighters said we should go with them. "We'll secure the bridge and this place and then you can go," they said. We saw some sense in this and did not want to take any more chances. We were scared to meet any government soldiers.

It was getting dark now and still raining hard. The fighters had walked in, but they wanted to leave. They asked Ben to help start some of the vehicles. One had a flat tire. Ben and Paul helped them change it, and we finally drove off back down the road the way we had come. We were the middle vehicle of three. It was pouring rain. We turned down another dirt road, and one of their vehicles broke down. They crammed all their men and guns and paraphernalia into the remaining two vehicles. Cathy sat on Monie's lap.

We arrived at a town called Vessy, where they had taken over a nice house for their headquarters. We all sat on a couch while they got a room ready for us. It was probably midnight by that time. I never saw so many guns in all my life as were in this dining and living room. They were telling their war stories about all the Krahn guys they had just killed. All of them had red cloth bands on their heads or wrists. They had layered clothes, like shorts over pants, socks over pant legs, and they were soaking wet. Yet they were all elated and bragging. They had successfully taken over Bo and stopped people escaping over the bridge. Later we heard that many Monrovia government families and officials had escaped into Sierra Leone before the Freedom Fighters arrived.

Finally, they gave us four ladies one room, and the guys another room. I was so glad to be out of the Freedom Fighters' sight. Two guys started to fight out there and someone broke it up. We finally calmed down somewhat. Safe, yet antsy. There was an indoor bathroom and some water in there to wash up a bit. We ate some soup out of a can. I slept on the floor and Monie, Cathy and Laura took the bed.

Later that night, they wanted our truck to deliver some "stuff" to the next town. Not wanting to lose our truck, Ben drove it for them rather than give them the key. He made two trips to Dia, which was the town we ended up staying at. We saw that our Land Cruisers (with SIM/ELWA printed on the doors) had been used all day to take families across the border to Sierra Leone. Later we heard that the Sierra Leone police on the other side of the bridge confiscated them from the Liberia soldiers and kept them for us.

In the morning, we were introduced to the CO (Commanding Officer) named Dixon. He was fairly friendly and said to us, "This place (Vessy) is not secure. Last night we found two soldiers hiding near here." And, of course, they killed them. He said we should move down to the next town (Dia) where it was secure and would be their headquarters in Cape Mount County.

As we were packing up and about to leave Vessy, I remember one of the fighters saying to me, "No bullet can enter me. We made good medicine, good medicine." They were loaded not just with weapons, but with juju (or medicine) for protection. Juju is an amulet or fetish believed to have a magic quality. And they were fearless. A nice Liberian lady come out of the house as we were leaving with rice and soup for us. By now we were hungry, having only snacked a bit all day Saturday and Sunday.

At Dia we stayed at a house with a nice Liberian family. On the way to Dia, Dixon had stopped at a place and came back with a live goat. He told the house family to cook it for us and gave them some rice. During that week they brought in four goats for us. I went out to the kitchen to sit with the woman who was cooking and got acquainted. They cooked the goat hide as well, so there were little hairs throughout the "gravy." I ate it, but some of our group were finding it too unappetizing.

While we were eating, one fighter came in and said, "We have a wounded man here. Can anybody help him?" Everybody looked at me. I said I would try. A bullet had gone right through his calf, missing the bones. He had country medicine on it and had it tied with a reed. I finally soaked all that off. I did not have any antiseptic, so I asked for some Clorox and diluted some in a cup. I washed the wound and he did not even wince. That was all I could do. I wanted to ask him, "What happened to your juju protection?", but I didn't dare. I gave him some erythromycin tabs and never saw him again. From then on, I was called "First Aid" by the Freedom Fighters.

On Tuesday, the only significant thing that happened was they found a government man and his wife hiding in town. They were taken out to the street. They begged for their lives and paid money. The fighters were shooting between their legs. Finally, they took them away to Robertsport on the coast. We were told on Tuesday that Sierra Leone had closed their border to everyone. Nobody could pass and we were stuck now. They said they informed their superiors in Robertsport about us and were waiting to hear from them with directions.

On Wednesday Ben started feeling sick. In the afternoon, Dixon came roaring into town and demanded to see Ben and told Ben they had found our other vehicles across the bridge at Sierra Leone (SL) police headquarters. SL police said they would give them only to Ben, so Ben should go with them now and collect them. But because Ben was sick, Paul went too. They actually walked over the bridge and talked with the SL police. They knew all about us. The SL police said Ben could take our two Land Cruisers, but Ben said he wanted them to keep the vehicles for him there. So the SL police declared the vehicles impounded, and thus Ben would be able to tell Dixon he could not get them after all.

Then a crucial thing happened. Ben saw a white woman across the road from the police station. He went to talk with her and discovered she was with the SL Red Cross. Ben explained everything and handed her a letter we had composed ahead of time, hoping to get it to someone who would tell our embassy we were alive but stranded. God gave us just the person to do that.

It was 9:30 p.m. before Ben and Paul got back to Dia. Ben was sicker than I had ever seen him with a fever of 104, chills, etc. I started him on quinine for five days for malaria treatment. By morning he could hardly hear due to side effects from quinine. Ben does not even remember that Thursday. We wondered if he had cerebral malaria.

Thursday was the longest day. Ben was out of it. Paul got real quiet and retreated to his room with Laura. I need to say that Paul made me very angry and upset that day when he showed me diamonds sewn into his underwear to sneak out of the country. That was illegal, and it put us all at great risk if he was caught with them. The rest of the week Paul stayed low key. Tim was real quiet. Monie would not let Cathy out of her sight. We had many short prayer meetings that day.

At the end of Thursday afternoon, a car whipped up in front of our house suddenly, and I said, "A white man just got out of that car!"

He walked into our house and said, "Hi! Man, I'm glad to see you guys. I'm Dean Eckert, Southern Baptist missionary. I used to work in this district with a well drilling machine."

The local people knew Dean very well. He had a Red Cross button on his bib jeans. He said he was here to help us. The Red Cross lady Ben and Paul talked with at the SL police station told Dean about us, and he bravely came over to Liberia and talked the rebels into driving him to us. Dean left and went to find Dixon. A miracle! Thank you, Lord. But Dean did not return that evening.

Early Friday morning CO Dixon said to pack up because he was taking us to Robertsport, a city on the coast. We all had to go. Paul agreed but I was not so sure. I became very upset with Liberia and all that was happening. There was no good reason to go to Robertsport when we should be going to Sierra Leone. I had been treating some sick people in town before this, but I stopped helping anybody in Liberia. And I found I was not afraid anymore either.

About 11 a.m. Dean drove in. I ran out and told him the fighters wanted to take us all to Robertsport. He said he would go on our behalf. He had an official reason to go because he needed to ask if the Red Cross could bring in some rice. Long story short, I think Dean made some kind of deal exchanging us for rice. He came back on Friday evening with a written pass for us to leave.

The pass granted us permission to move from Dia back to the main road at Tiene, six miles from the bridge and Bo. Dean was exhausted, having run back to us at Dia, so we fed him. He insisted we leave that night, though. I wondered and still wonder what Dean knew and did not tell us. We all had the suspicion that someone wanted to demand ransom for our release.

Dean was working under the hood of one car to take us out when the whole place went berserk. The fighters starting shooting in the air and shouting in victory because Charles Taylor announced on ELWA radio he had taken over the government and was now the CIC (Commander-in-Chief). They started driving vehicles up and down and celebrating. With Charles Taylor taking control of ELWA and all the "celebrating" going on, we could not leave.

We got up early on Saturday. Dean insisted we really must leave, but there wasn't a car around. Although Ben was feeling much better from his malaria bout, he did not have the strength to walk to Tiene. Even Monie and Laura could not have walked. It would be about ten miles out to the main road at Tiene. Finally, Dean, Tim and Cathy, myself, and a Liberian were going to walk, and the rest would catch up as soon as they could secure a car. We were just about to leave when a brand-new black Mercedes drove into town. Dean talked to the driver. He read our pass and agreed to take some of us and our hand luggage. I never saw my suitcase again. It was left at Dia. The car had come back and got those of us who had walked about three miles.

At Tiene they showed us a room to wait in that was near the CO office. Lots of foot traffic, arguing, and guns surrounded us. We needed a spokesperson. Paul said he thought he was getting malaria. Ben was there, but he could hardly hear anything due to the side effects of quinine. So I became our spokesperson to get us out. If there is such a thing as righteous anger, I had it, and God used this for good. I was determined and totally unafraid.

Dean had finally found Dixon in Tiene. He read our pass and noted it only said we could go to Tiene. So Dixon and Sam, another CO, said they would send a runner to Robertsport and ask what to do with us now. Dean took off for Sierra Leone and came back with a bag of rice, some sugar, three gallons of gasoline, and cigarettes. He gave it to Dixon and Sam and kept telling them he wanted to bring in some Red Cross rice. Everyone knew that Dean meant in exchange for our release. I wanted to find some medicine in the trunk of the black Mercedes for Paul, but we had no idea where the car was. Paul and Laura and I went out looking for the car. We found it way across town, where I found Dean. By that time my righteous anger had kicked in high gear. I was determined we were leaving today and here it was afternoon already.

I told Dean I could not go back and sit in that little room again. What I did not tell him was that one of the bad Freedom Fighters had threatened me with rape when he returned from wherever he was going. I needed some privacy, a bathroom, and some supplies. Moni was exhausted and worried. Cathy was crying a lot. Ben was trying to rest in a chair. Tim was reading a book nonstop. Paul was getting sicker. We were all at our wits' end.

I said, "Come on, Dean, we are going to talk to Dixon and Sam." I was not afraid one bit. With God's help, I was going to talk us out of Liberia.

Meanwhile, ELWA came back on the air, and Charles Taylor announced four of his ministers of government. There was more shooting in celebration in Tiene. Dean and I arrived where Dixon and Sam were, near the room where everyone else was waiting.

I said to Dixon, "We are leaving Liberia. I will not sleep in Liberia again. There is fighting in the house and it is no place for visitors. What would Charles Taylor say if he saw our group sick and hungry and two having a nervous breakdown? We are ELWA missionaries and we need to leave now." I really laid it on heavy and determined and did so with no fear.

Dean explained that what the pass meant was that we were to go to Tiene, and then the COs would decide when was the right time and way for us to go. He convinced them that they were to decide what to do with us. Finally, Dixon said all right.

He ordered two cars and told us to get in. Four of us got in the back of the one car, and four of us in the back of the other. Dixon got in the front of the one with the driver. Sam and Dean got in the front of the other with its driver. We sped out of Tiene and Dixon kept telling the driver to go faster. Dean told us later that they were expecting some government soldiers around Bo that day and some fighting. Dixon had his gun ready, out the window, ready to shoot, during the six miles to Bo and the bridge.

When we arrived at the bridge, a Freedom Fighter saluted Dixon and took his weapons. I was surprised that Dixon was going to cross the bridge with us. He did and he talked with the SL policeman and handed us over. The car with Sam and Dean and the others was slower.

We could not see them and were beginning to worry, but finally they came over the bridge as well.

We were out. We were finally free.

We had nothing but what was in our pockets. I had a Kleenex and a copy of my passport pinned in my pocket. We felt great . . . safe . . . free . . . alive . . . hungry. In all the excitement, none of us noticed that Dean got back in the car with Dixon and went back across the bridge. The policeman saw this. Dean went back and got all our bags in the trunk of that black Mercedes.

While we were waiting for Dean to come back, the nice Sierra Leone policemen gave us MREs (Meals Ready to Eat), which were left over from the Middle East military, they said. They tasted so good. By the grace of God, we had our two Land Cruisers at the police station because Ben had told them to keep them for us. The SL police sent a Morse code message to all checkpoints en route to Freetown (the capital of Sierra Leone), clearing our way to travel without passports. We started driving that Saturday night to the Red Cross station where Dean was working in SL. We arrived well after midnight. Some kind people put us up for the rest of the night. We even got to take a bucket bath in the morning. We drove all day Sunday and arrived in Freetown late Sunday night.

We stayed with the Assembly of God missionaries in Freetown. It was all so overwhelming. Someone had a ham radio in Freetown, and we called SIM headquarters. They were relieved and ordered everyone to come home as soon as possible. No discussion. At 2:00 p.m. on Monday we had a debriefing meeting at the American embassy. They heard our account of what happened. They put a rush on getting us new passports. They asked us if we needed anything. I said I needed to call my family, but they would not let us use their communications to call home. The State Department in Washington DC called my parents and told them I was out of Liberia and safe. Of course, SIM had already called my parents.

I had a new passport and ticket home within three days. KLM gave me credit to purchase a ticket. I was to turn in this ticket invoice to SIM immediately upon arriving in the U.S. and make payment to KLM. We did, and I never forgot KLM's kindness to me for that ticket home. I really had no accessible money.

It was not until I reached Brussels airport that I could call home. I did not care and did not know what time it was in Michigan. I called home and assured my family I was all right, but there was going to be a lot of explaining to do! I was the first one of us to get to SIM headquarters in Charlotte, NC. Ben and Monie arrived shortly after. I did not see Paul and Laura again after we got to Freetown. I spent a few days at SIM headquarters and finally flew home to Hadley on August 4. By the grace of God we were unharmed and home. My status with SIM was "home for special reasons." I was not on furlough and not on field assignment. That status would last for seven months.

Of note is that only two weeks after I got home, I had to go back to North Carolina. The Mission called all Liberia missionaries to a one week gathering at Ridgecrest Baptist Conference for a retreat. We all had bits and pieces of the story. It needed to be told and heard by all. That was a wise move by Larry Fehl and Gerry Johnson to organize this wonderful reunion. About 140 people were there, including about 60 kids. My mother, Lee Warsen, and I drove from Michigan to attend the retreat in late August 1990. There were three main goals: (1) to be spiritually renewed by asking the Lord what now, and asking the Lord to help us overcome fears and resentment against Liberia's government; (2) for first-hand accounts of what happened so we all had the complete story "from the horses' mouth";(3) to get an outlook of the prospects of returning to Liberia to work. Counselors were available and a speaker talked about signs of stress.

Jon Shea (Liberia director) reported to us that on July 5 our American embassy told him that Charles Taylor sent a message saying we should not have people in the transmitter building. So a decision was made to shut down ELWA transmitters. ELWA radio had been broadcasting for thirty-six years straight without missing a day. He cried.

I told everyone of our harrowing eight days with the rebels and how we finally managed to get out. So many touching and nerve-wracking accounts were shared that week. Our joy over a safe departure and being reunited with our families was marred by a deep sense of loss and our concern for Liberian friends left behind.

To close, I want to quote an article from SIM *Intercom,* October-November 1990 issue:

"What showed up as most important to SIM during the crisis in Liberia? It wasn't property, equipment, or programs. It was people.

During the conflict, we assured Jon Shea, Western Africa Area Director, that we agreed with him on that. The safety of our missionaries and Liberian staff was more important to us than protection of any property. Jon and Pat Shea and eight other SIMers stayed on at the ELWA compound, crowded with 22,000 displaced persons, because their presence staved off the tribal killings taking place outside the compound. When they saw that their presence was no longer a deterrent to violence they left, but not without taking several wounded Liberians with them. As to personal possessions, including irreplaceable family mementos, they simply walked away from them. Jon Shea's last act, before heading for the border, was to dispense an advance in pay to every Liberian staffer he could find."

Not only had I come home empty handed, I found I had very few belongings at home either. I had taken most of my summer clothes to Liberia. I remember being invited to a youth group swim party and having to decline because I did not have a swimsuit. So I went to Hurley Hospital in Flint, Michigan, got an interview with the head nurse of their Emergency Room (ER), and she hired me! I was upfront with her about going back to Africa in a few months, but that didn't seem to matter. I was grateful for the job.

Working in the ER at this city hospital was a dream come true and I liked it. I spent everything I made replacing my wardrobe for when I was able to return overseas. I also bought a ham radio and started taking amateur radio lessons while making plans to join the Sierra Leone team. The Kuwait war occurred in January and February, 1991, which delayed our plans to go to Sierra Leone, but not for long. Sierra Leone and then Ethiopia were temporary assignments while I waited for Liberia to settle down.

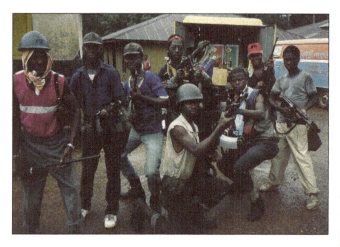

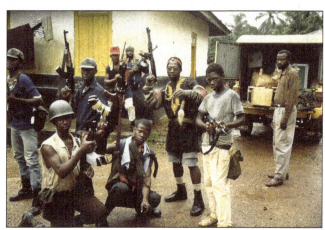

These two pictures are of the proud Liberian Freedom Fighters we were "with" for seven days. Ben Motis took these pictures.

Six of us who were detained at the border, plus Dean:

Tim Motis
Dean Ekberg
Monie Motis
Me
Paul (Laura is taking the picture)
Cathy Motis
A Liberian
Ben Motis

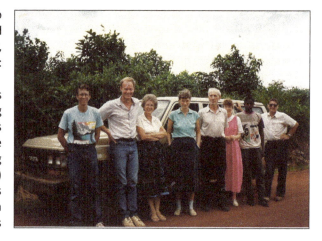

# SIM Missionary Tells of Getting Caught in Liberian Cross-fire

It may shock many Americans to know that their fellow countrymen are prevented from leaving Iraq and Kuwait or that others were forcefully detained in Liberia.

Barb Hartwig would not be surprised. She knows what it's like to be detained overseas.

Before she fled Liberia July 28, she and six other Americans were captives of first one band of soldiers and then another. For a time they were caught in cross-fire between opposing forces while barricaded behind furniture in a customs office.

Miss Hartwig was in the last group of SIM missionaries to leave Liberia. In an interview at the headquarters of her mission at Charlotte, N.C., she told *World* about two harrowing months of trying to stay clear of that West African country's internal strife.

She and Mr. and Mrs. Ben Motis were stationed at Tahn in Grand Cape Mount Country, near the border of Sierra Leone, when SIM officials decided in late May

that it would be advisable for them to go to a safer location. Tahn was on a main route leading to Monrovia, the embattled capital city, and there was speculation that troops would come through on their way to Monrovia. SIM didn't want its church planting team caught there in a possible standoff between troops loyal to President Samuel Doe and those of the opposing National Patriotic Front (NPLF).

So the Motises (and their college age son, Tim, and daughter, Cathy, who had just come "home" for the summer) and Miss Hartwig took off for Kolahun, up in the corner of the country, near the point at which Guinea, Sierra Leone and Liberia meet. They were there with other missionaries through much of June, but then hostilities threatened in that area. The team headed back to Tahn to say farewell to Liberian co-workers, to pack up what they could take out of the country and to make final arrangements for securing the mission property.

## Leaving not easy

Leaving the site of their work July 21 was not easy. The team had organized nine congregations in and around Tahn. Leaders were developing, and the missionaries had been training them with theological education by extension courses. Miss Hartwig had worked in community health and had trained nurse-midwives. She had seen the rate of deaths fall dramatically through an inoculation program. In addition to her medical activities she had taught the Bible (officially "religious knowledge" classes) in junior high in government schools.

Curfew and the hazards of taking vehicles into the bush prevented team members from holding worship services at all of the points at which they

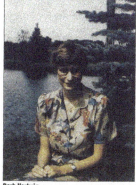

**Barb Hartwig**

worked, but she reported that they were able to pray with a number of the believers before they left.

"I love them," she said of the Liberian Christians left behind. "They're like family."

Miss Hartwig told *World* that she assured her students that they would remember what she had taught them and that "nobody can take it away from you."

With the Motises and Miss Hartwig when they left Tahn was an American Christian couple who had been working there under a Liberian mining license, seeking minerals in a nearby river.

## Passports seized

The party of seven arrived in Bo, a town near the border with Sierra Leone Saturday evening (July 21), only to be told by government troops that they must turn in their U.S. passports and their vehicle registration documents. Furthermore, the fleeing Americans were warned not to leave town "on orders from the mansion" (meaning President Samuel Doe's presidential headquarters in Monrovia).

"We slept in the cars" that night, Miss Hartwig related. A rumor of approaching rebel forces cause a stampede of the indigenous population, but the Americans were ordered at gunpoint not to leave.

The troops guarding them were nervous as Sunday (July 22) dawned. Their trigger fingers were at the ready, and Miss Hartwig declared, "it was our worst day." At 5:30 p.m. the NPLF did invade. The Americans got behind a barricade of fur-

**Camp guard:** *A young woman guards rebel refugees late last week while waiting for a pass to leave the squalid Liberian camp where more than 200,000 people had gathered to escape the bitter fighting which has gone on for months.* [AP]

An article in the World magazine (August 25, 1990, issue)

niture in the customs post as shooting broke out.

"Not one shell came in," the missionary recalled of their hiding place. "It was a miracle."

Motis hailed one of the invaders and identified himself as an American missionary, and to his relief the response was, "We're freedom fighters, here to protect you."

### Still detained

That "protection," however, amounted to continued detention. Even though the small party was very near a river crossing into Sierra Leone, the NPLF commander said he was not able to allow them to depart.

At that point, a Southern Baptist missionary, Dean Ekberg, appeared as part of a Red Cross relief contingent based at Zimi, Sierra Leone. Ekberg, who otherwise spent his time drilling wells and providing water supplies, interceded and finally got permission from the NPLF district commander at Robertsport for the seven to leave.

They had been awaiting that permission for nearly a week when the Americans walked across the Mano River bridge at 6 p.m., July 28. They walked because their vehicles had been confiscated, but when they reached the border post on the Sierra Leone side the guards handed them the keys to an SIM vehicle. Troops fleeing the conflict had tried to drive it into the neighboring country, but officials there saw that it was mission property and held it for the missionaries. (Only the smallest pieces of their luggage were returned.)

### Freetown freedom

They got into Freetown, the capital of Sierra Leone, at 2 p.m., Monday, June 30, where Assembly of God missionaries provided hospitality and assistance with the next steps of their journey. Their passports had never been returned, so the AOG hosts took them to the consul's office at the U.S. embassy and started the process of getting replacements. They also got them reservations on flights to Europe and then home.

The new passports were prepared quickly. Miss Hartwig's new one has an expiration date of July 30, 2000. Her mission is committed to the cooperative "World by 2000" international evangelization effort, and the passport will serve until that year.     —A.H.M.

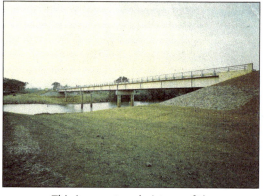

This is a postcard picture of the Mano River Bridge between Liberia and Sierra Leone. Seven of us were detained for eight days on the Liberia side in July, 1990.

This article is used by courtesy of *The Flint Journal*, August 10, 1990.

# ETRO

## D1

☐ CLASSIFIED, D4
☐ WEATHER, D12

THE FLINT JOURNAL • FRIDAY, AUGUST 10, 1990

# Cookies free captives

## Lapeer woman held seven days in Liberia

By EDWARD L. RONDERS
Journal Lapeer Bureau

HADLEY TWP. — Chocolate chip cookies helped secure freedom for seven Americans, including a Lapeer County native, who were held captive for seven days last month by Liberian rebels.

Barbara Hartwig, a 1973 Lapeer High School graduate, found herself looking down the barrel of an AK-47 and later dodging bullets while government troops battled invading rebels.

When the shooting stopped early July 22, Hartwig and the other six Americans were among the rebels. So Hartwig and her group appealed to their sweet tooth.

"The freedom fighters saw our triple batch of chocolate chip cookies, and they loved them," she said in her parents' Hadley Township farmhouse.

"The cookies seemed to reassure them we were friendly Americans.

They told us to feel free. But that was hard to do with shooting still going on."

Hartwig, a 34-year-old missionary with the Sudan Interior Mission, an interdenominational mission agency, became entangled in the West African civil war while on a missionary assignment to Tahn in northwest Liberia.

Less than two days after the rebels freed Hartwig and the others, government troops stormed a Lutheran church in the Liberian capital of Monrovia, about 80 miles away, and killed an estimated 600 people who had sought refuge there.

Liberia, a country founded by freed U.S. slaves that became a republic in 1847, has been wracked by unrest for eight months, as rebels try to oust President Samuel Doe.

The U.S. State Department had warned Americans to leave the country earlier and offered to evacuate them,

but Hartwig remained, feeling secure until late July.

"The embassy can only recommend you leave the country," she said. "We're under the direction of the SIM, and they, like the embassy, kept a skeleton staff in Liberia. It was my choice to stay."

Hartwig said her captivity was more a case of bad timing than anything else.

She said she was with two other missionaries and their two children when they decided to leave the West African country.

After securing their mission in Tahn, they set out for Bo, a village on the Sierra Leone border. Along the way, they picked up two more Americans, who had been working in the diamond fields.

But when they reached a bridge at the Sierra Leone border, they were told

**Please see CAPTIVE — D3**

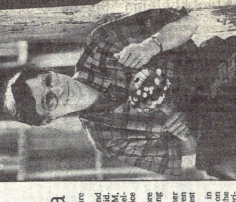

JOURNAL PHOTO/KENT MILLER

Barbara Hartwig found herself staring down the barrel of an AK-47 rifle while being held captive in Liberia.

# CAPTIVE

**CONTINUED FROM D1**

they could not leave the country.

The Americans pooled their money and offered it to the soldiers, who took it and nodded approval for them to leave. But another soldier stationed in the middle of the bridge was not in on the deal.

"He looked at us, pointed his gun right at us and said, 'No, go back.' I put the Landcruiser in reverse right away," Hartwig said.

The group took refuge in a Liberian customs office, where they built a barricade using desks, an old freezer and anything else they could find.

At 5:30 the next morning, gunfire erupted just after Hartwig had brushed her teeth.

"We literally dived behind that barricade when the shooting started," she said. "We could hear bullets hitting the building and glass breaking all around."

None of the Americans ventured outside when the shooting diminished. Instead, they yelled out that they were American missionaries in hopes that the rebels were friendly.

The rebels cautiously approached the group, but the chocolate chip cookies convinced the soldiers that they meant no harm, Hartwig said.

The Americans were taken to Dhia, a village about 15 miles from the border, but they were uncertain if they were free to go.

Their break came when they gave a letter detailing their plight to a woman from the Red Cross who was visiting the area. The letter eventually found its way to Dean Ekberg, a Southern Baptist missionary in Sierra Leone.

Ekberg crossed the border, found Hartwig's group and tried to negotiate their release, offering hard-to-get gasoline and cigarettes.

"He went to the commander of the rebels in Robertsport on the coast and got permission to move us to another town," Hartwig said. "But once we got there, we were told we had to be moved to Robertsport. The commander wanted to see us."

Hartwig had a sinking feeling the rebels were about to begin using their captives for political gain. Overcome with frustration, she said she let the rebels know her feelings in no uncertain terms.

"The one local commander said we would have to sleep in that village another night," Hartwig said. "Well, I was not going to spend one more night in Liberia. I looked him right in the eye and said, 'No!'"

Finally, after seven days in captivity, two rebels put them into their cars and escorted them into Sierra Leone.

Hartwig said she plans to stay in Lapeer County until the political climate stabilizes in the strife-torn country.

Once that happens, though, she plans on going back — with an ample supply of chocolate chip cookies, of course.

Reunion at the airport with my parents!

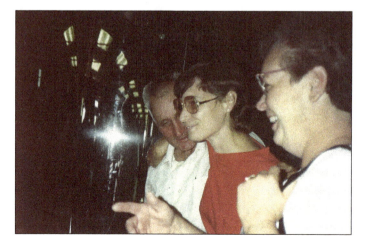

## CHAPTER 7

# IN FREETOWN, SIERRA LEONE FOR LIBERIA (1991–92)

*On March 4,* 1991, I arrived in Freetown, Sierra Leone (SL). I had been home for seven months to recuperate from our ordeal in escaping from Liberia. SIM had never had ministry work in this country before. A handful of missionaries, including me, received a one-year assignment in Freetown because the United Nations started daily relief flights between Freetown and Monrovia, Liberia. SIM/ELWA missionaries were qualified as relief workers in Liberia, so we could use these free flights. It was my privilege and joy to enable many relief workers, not just SIMers, to connect with the daily flight service to Monrovia and those returning from Monrovia. John Corey, Pat O'Neil, and I rented a big house with seven large bedrooms, a large dining room, a sitting room, and a kitchen. Ten days after we arrived, we moved in and then worked hard and fast to clean and set up the bedrooms with curtains, beds, mosquito nets, bedding, and furniture. I also set up accounting for our guests and for the relief work we would be doing. I had to keep the guesthouse money separate from relief work money, plus keep my personal money separate. Our first "guests" arrived shortly after we moved in; Ben Motis was among them. God bless Ben. I remember he helped me get a water system set up the weekend before he flew out to Monrovia. He was one of the first to return to Monrovia and see the devastation at ELWA.

What did my parents think of my return? I promised them that I would not go back into Liberia that year. I promised to remain in Sierra Leone to support those who were returning. And I kept my word to them. Some tried to talk me into returning to Liberia to help, too, but this time I was "holding the rope." Little did I know when I went to Freetown how Liberians were going to come to me there!

Others came temporarily to help in Sierra Leone during those fourteen months of operating the house we had rented, which we called Bethany House, but I stayed from start to finish of our rent agreement. Bethany was the name of the village where Jesus stayed with Mary and Martha and Lazarus in the Bible, so I nicknamed our guest house after that village near Jerusalem. It proved to be what I still think was the best and most useful work and ministry I did during all my time in Africa. My years in South Sudan ran a close second.

Every day was full of new challenges. I had to run a guest house with no refrigerator or oven due to no electricity. I could have cried when I tried and tried to find where to light the gas inside the oven, only to find out it was an electric oven with gas stove burners. For one year, I pretty much made one of three desserts cooked on the gas stove burners: either custard, or homemade chocolate syrup to serve on cut bananas with peanuts, or no-bake chocolate oatmeal cookies. Eventually we set up breakfast on a do-it-yourself basis. I kept all the makings for a self-help breakfast in one big cupboard. Guests were to help themselves to whatever they wanted for breakfast. I hired a Liberian named Irving to prepare our mid-day meal six days a week. He would go to the market every day and buy ingredients for Liberian "rice and soup," which he then cooked. Irving would serve the cooked food in metal dishes with covers that kept just fine for two or three hours while guests came in to eat lunch. We had no way to keep leftovers, but nothing went to waste, as we always found someone to finish it up. Irving's brother Kollie did all the laundry and cleaning at Bethany House.

For a while I was trying to cook the evening meal for everyone, but it was too much. We went full swing into the refugee camp work. I gave every guest directions to different local restaurants to choose from, or they could go down the street to a small grocery store if they preferred to cook something simple for themselves for supper. It worked very smoothly for everyone. On Sunday, I did cook for everyone. Usually it was spaghetti. With such a rapid turnover of guests, the short menu options and repetition of menu only affected those of us who lived at Bethany House. Randy and Adena Wildman helped with logistics in Bethany House for a while, but they eventually went on into Liberia, and Pete and Sadie Ackley came to help run Bethany House for a while.

The Southern Baptist Mission in Freetown had been "babysitting" our two Land Cruisers while we were gone, so it was great to have vehicles for use in Freetown. One of the best decisions we made was to hire Issa Kargbo, a Sierra Leonean, to be our general business helper. He taught me to navigate Freetown roads, where to buy things in stores, and how to exchange money to the Leone currency.

How did we know who was coming and going to Liberia via Freetown? It was all by amateur (ham) radio communications. While "home-for-special reasons" the previous six months, I had studied amateur radio lessons and Morse code for my general amateur license because I knew it would be essential to operations in Freetown. John Corey was a ham operator too, and he set up my antenna on the roof of Bethany House. With my US amateur license in hand, I had my Sierra Leone license to operate as 9L1LP on just my second day in Sierra Leone. I started operating immediately using a solar-powered battery on the floor. We call that running barefoot (without an amplifier). I had a good signal around the world and it was fun. I also did radio "patches" for anyone who needed to call home. Every morning I called in to ELWA station folks. And every late afternoon I called Ron Sonius or someone else in the U.S. for information on who was coming and going. Randy or Pete or someone else made a lot of trips on the ferry boat to Freetown's international airport across the bay to receive our guests. To make an international phone call in Freetown in 1991, one had to stand in a long line at the downtown telecommunications building. I still had to do that many times because "money business" could not be conducted via ham radio, and I handled the SIM Project money that ran our S.L. operations.

Just to complicate life a little more, on March 23, Liberian rebels crossed the border into Sierra Leone and attacked and captured two main towns in southern S.L. They raided for food and goods. We did not know if their intent included a political agenda. Charles Taylor denied involvement in it. Long story short, they got up to the Kenema area. I resolved not to meet "those guys" again! I kept a close ear to daily BBC radio reports about the rebels' progress. The SL army did manage to contain them outside Kenema for a long time. But all of that activity along the border with Liberia caused a sudden influx of Liberian refugees to the Freetown area. The UN set up a refugee camp on an old airstrip at Waterloo, twenty miles outside of Freetown. Issa and Randy Wildman and Pete Ackley and I started going out there immediately to help. At its peak, about 8,000 Liberians came to Waterloo to escape the fighting along the border of SL and Liberia. We drove out there every Monday, Wednesday, and Friday to teach, visit, listen, and pray with families. The majority of them were women and children. Most of the women did not know where their husbands were, or else they were already widowed. Knowing Liberian English made me an accepted and a welcome worker among them. I even knew many who came from our Gola district. I was known as Yomo, my given Gola name.

I made it my work to eventually visit every single "tent" family in the camp. I looked for needs that I could come back and help with. I held a clothes drive in Freetown and took bags of clothes to the camp. I did my work quietly going tent by tent. No one asked any of the refugees which tribe they were from. For some, I simply read a Bible portion each time I went to visit. Many had money and would give me money to buy a certain item for them in Freetown. The refugee camp UN authorities only asked that we not give food. So I did not get involved in any food distribution. One day I was walking down the center airstrip, and a UN vehicle stopped me and accused me of handing out food. I showed him I only had empty jars in my bag to give out, no food.

The Red Cross ran a clinic for the refugees, but it had limited medicines, so sometimes I could bring a select medicine to someone. I remember entering a tent one day and finding a woman who had just delivered twins. She was a new mother and I showed her how to breastfeed her babies. And I asked a kind, motherly "neighbor" woman to visit her for support. One day I was invited into a tent where an old man was dying. I sat with the family for a while and then I asked how I could help. They wanted me to bathe him. So I did and left everything as tidy as I could. All the while I was giving a word of testimony for the Lord to the family.

I never knew when I arrived on a given day what I would find in my visits. One man I visited was regretting the loss of his barbering tools. Issa managed to get him some, and he was elated to start up his trade again as a barber. As a team we organized a Christian concert one weekend that everyone seemed to enjoy. A certain NGO (non-government organization) set up a school, and I helped them with school supplies.

One day I saw some newcomers, women, sitting under a big tree weaving fishing nets. I had learned from our traditional birth attendants in Liberia how to do this. I greeted the women, sat on the ground with them, and just took the net from one woman's hands and started weaving it. They were shocked that I knew how to do it! We talked about fishing. I had been fishing in rivers with women who netted their catch. Only men fished with a fishing pole. All my culture learning at Tahn paid dividends that culminated in the refugee camp ministry.

One cannot measure the spiritual impact of that year of refugee camp work. I did the best I could to talk about spiritual things, read the Bible, and pray with folks who were willing. What a privilege to be there that year with the background to make a difference in many people's lives during a sad period of history. "Yomo and Issa" made a good team out there. Issa and his wife, Daphne, are heading up the "Christians in Action" mission in Freetown today. I support them and the tough church development work they are carrying on in Sierra Leone.

One day I looked at my personal SIM account statement and saw a new supporter listed with an address in Alaska. I knew no one in Alaska, so I wrote to them and asked how they knew me. They said that someone from International Military Ministries was at their church as a guest speaker. This missionary to soldiers gave a sermon illustration from my work in Freetown. Apparently, we had given them rooms at Bethany House. This family found out how to support the missionary he spoke of in his sermon. From then on they supported me. I never saw or talked with them. I just knew them through correspondence. It's a small world sometimes.

Another small world account was the day I happened to visit some United Methodist missionaries in Freetown. When I was invited in and they heard my name, they asked me if I knew any Hartwigs in Flint, because a Bob Hartwig had done their wedding photos many years ago. I said, "Yes, that was my Uncle Bob and Aunt June!" What a cool connection with home. They helped me get in touch with a surgeon at their United Methodist (UM) Eye Hospital in Freetown. The ELWA missionaries in Monrovia wanted to send a young boy my way who needed an eye operation due to a terrible BB gun accident that had blinded him in one eye. Michael came to Freetown and had the operation at the United Methodist Eye Hospital. I held his hand throughout the operation, as he was so scared, and then took care of him at Bethany House for a few weeks. He was and is a gifted pianist who played by ear and eventually made it from Liberia to the U.S. to live.

One day I had a visit from people from the Lutheran Mission in Freetown who had started a school for about 120 Liberian street kids. They asked me to come and assess the kids for health needs and visit them regularly at the school. I was torn between knowing I should help, but wondering how to do more. Issa said he knew of a SL nurse named Zena who we could hire to do this work. I met Zena and she was/is a wonderful Christian nurse. We went together on Thursday mornings to this school. First, we identified those who were undernourished, and they began receiving extra food from the school. At first almost every child needed some kind of medicine. Zena bought all the medicines and followed up on each child as needed. I only had to go on Thursday mornings and assess the children. Eventually hardly any child was left with a chronic condition.

I remember asking for and getting the opportunity to do CEF (Child Evangelism Fellowship) lessons in class. It was great. Training a national person to do the work is how to make one's work sustainable and how to get more done. Zena continued on at this school in Freetown for a long time, plus she came out to the refugee camp with us sometimes for ministry needs. I cannot say enough about how wonderful and important both Issa and Daphne, and Joshua and Zena were in our work that year. Some years later, Zena and Joshua and their two boys came to Ghana to attend Bible College in Accra. They came up to Tamale and stayed with me between Christmas Day and New Year's Day three times, as I recall.

Another opportunity came my way in Freetown. I already mentioned our daily cook, a Liberian named Irving. Irving's brother Kollie was Bethany House's cleaner and laundry helper. These brothers were good basketball players and asked me to sponsor a basketball team they were assembling for a tournament coming up. They said all I would have to do is sign a paper as sponsor and pay for the T-shirts for the team. I couldn't say no. I agreed. Grace, a young Liberian friend in Freetown, also a refugee, and I went to the games and cheered them on to victory! They won! It was all very exciting. This Liberian team beat the SL teams and Lebanese team in the tournament. I gave team devotions a couple of times. Again, its impact is not measurable this side of heaven.

Our twelve-month lease on Bethany House was extended about a month, but finally SIM said to wrap up our work there and close the guesthouse. The daily UN flights to Monrovia from Freetown had stopped because flights could now fly straight to downtown Monrovia. The refugee camp work was endless. Lee Sonius came to Freetown and helped me close up Bethany House. We packed a forty-foot container with a Land Cruiser and household goods to ship to Monrovia for use at ELWA. For the last two or three weeks or so, I stayed with some single missionary friends in the neighborhood. Now it came down to my last day in Freetown. I had a ticket home on KLM the next day. I was packed and planned to spend my last day at the beach just relaxing, but that day we woke up to the sounds of gunfire in the city. Oh, no!

Let me quote from my June 1992 prayer letter. "My April 30 KLM ticket was in hand when 'it' started at 8:15 a.m. on the 29. I heard this message on a two-meter radio from our American embassy consular: "Attention all stations: do not come downtown. There is a major shoot-out at government buildings right now. Everybody should go home immediately and lock your doors!"

A group of soldiers had begun a protest at the State House in downtown Freetown. Support built up and the protest turned into a coup as the president finally escaped SL on April 30. We stayed indoors for three days and followed events on our local radio network, including USA embassy reports and BBC broadcasts. I felt fairly secure with my friends, but actually we expected soldiers to come to the door and demand the key to our vehicles, but the knock never came. We heard gunfire very close, and at one point we had to take our Scrabble game to the floor one afternoon, but nothing happened at our house, praise the Lord.

By the grace of God, I had sold my ham radio to a Lebanese man just the night before the coup. That was the last bit of business I had needed to conduct. My plan was to use that personal sale money to go home and purchase another radio. Had I not sold it, I would have just left it behind, and never seen it again or received any compensation for it.

The American embassy in SL announced an evacuation plan for American citizens who wanted to leave. Though it was a relatively bloodless coup, the embassy said this may be the lull before the storm. The airport was closed as well as all businesses. I was grateful for a safe and immediate way to get out and go home. I signed up to go.

My parents received this second call, within one year, from our State Department saying, "Your daughter is fine and coming home." Oh, great. I really did not feel in much danger, but my family did not understand what all was going on. A group of Green Berets stationed in Germany and an Air Force crew with a C130 plane came to the Freetown airport. About 450 Americans were lined up to leave. My passport was stamped as valid for only one year until or unless I paid for this evacuation. We were not informed of how much it would cost, or where they were taking us! You just sign on the dotted line that you will pay and be dropped off somewhere. I went. We were all taken to Dakar, Senegal, to the north, where we were left in the care of one hotel to sort out the rest of our journey to wherever we wanted to go. Well, KLM does not fly in Senegal. But Sabena Airlines did and they honored my KLM ticket home! Hurrah. This time I had a credit card with me and I needed it to pay my hotel bill. After not having a credit card when I needed one to leave Liberia via Guinea, I made sure I never came to Africa again without a credit card, and here I was already using it.

I spent about four days in Dakar sorting out my ticket home. A bunch of us were at a nice hotel on the coast, and we enjoyed our time there very much. On our second day, we were surprised one afternoon at the pool when some of the same American Green Berets who had evacuated us came in and joined us! They were given a day's leave or something and were anxious to hear our story about the coup. They bought us a Coke and wanted to find some souvenirs and gifts for their wives. We helped them get some nice things from a market. As it turned out, I traded my Freetown T-shirt for one of the guy's military Bible. I still have it. I agreed to do it when he promised me he could and would replace it.

A little trend was forming here. I reflected on the fact that this was the third time I had experienced a sudden unexpected "event" on the eve of a trip home from Africa. In Benin, the thieves had entered our house at night and stole my purse from my bedside. In Liberia, Ben and Monie and I were not expecting trouble at the SL border that day because our Wesleyan friends had exited that border just the day before with no trouble. Now the coup happened the day before I was to leave Freetown. Okay, Lord. You know what is best.

I made it home the day before Mother's Day and cooked dinner for my whole family on Mother's Day! Wow. What a year!

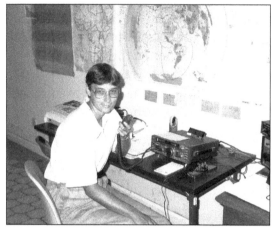

While in Freetown, I had daily morning radio contact with ELWA in Liberia to coordinate travelers.

In the evenings, I had amateur radio contact with Ron Sonius and others to coordinate those coming to Liberia via Freetown.

My call sign was 9L1LP in Sierra Leone.
My USA call sign is N8NMU.

Standing with Issa Kargbo at Waterloo Refugee Camp. Issa is a Sierra Leoneon pastor who was tremendously helpful with all the refugee business and Freetown business. I am holding Matthew, whose mother died in the war. Older folks are often left to raise their grandchildren.

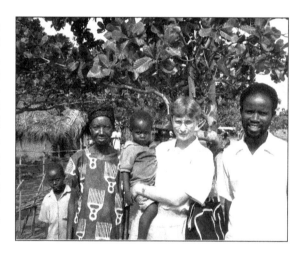

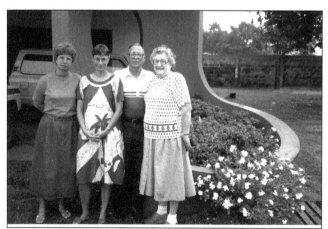

Pete and Sadie Ackley and Renate Isert ( SIM missionaries too) were living at Bethany House and helping with logistics and refugee camp work in 1991.

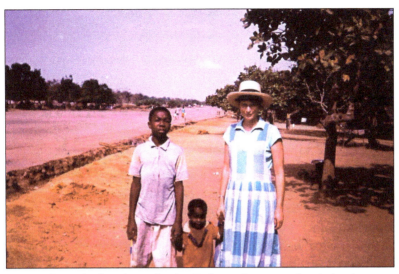

The United Nations Liberian Refugee Camp was located outside Freetown at an old airstrip site. About 8,000 Liberians
eventually occupied this camp.

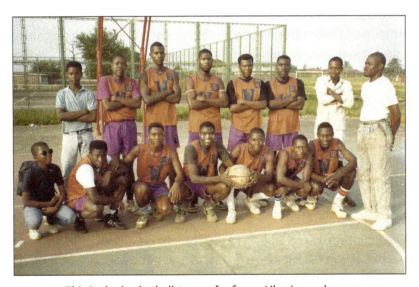

This is the basketball team of refugee Liberians who won
a tournament. The one holding the basketball and team
captain is Irving, our guest house cook almost every day.
And Kollie is the first one standing on the right side who
was our house laundry and cleaning helper. Grace and I
are not pictured, but she and I went to all the games and
cheered them on!

CHAPTER 8

# SUMMARY OF THE CIVIL WAR IN LIBERIA AND EBOLA OUTBREAK

*Charles Taylor and* his Freedom Fighters, (also known as rebels or National Patriotic Front of Liberia), started the tribal war on Christmas Eve, 1989. Taylor was from a certain tribe we will not mention and tried to take over the government from Samuel Doe, who had become Commander-in-Chief of Liberia in a bloody 1980 coup. Taylor and his rebels entered Liberia from Ivory Coast and slowly fought their way to the capital city, Monrovia. It is said that this civil war started as a tribal conflict, but it quickly turned into an economic "war" as Taylor eventually exploited the natural resources of Liberia, such as gold, diamonds, timber, and iron ore.

It was truly a volatile situation in 1990 and 1991 and periodically afterwards. President Samuel Doe was caught, tortured, and killed not by Taylor, but by another warlord and his followers. West African peacekeepers entered Monrovia, and the warring factors accepted a cease-fire. It was all complicated by the warlords who popped up vying for power and government. I am not even going to try to name all those factions or explain this terrible civil war that set Liberia back about a hundred years! The Gola tribe was not one of the primary warring tribes.

Did I ever return to Liberia? I did for two weeks in 1996. You know the saying, if you fall off a horse, get up and get back on. I did not want the difficult eight days of being detained at the border to be my last experience in Liberia. I decided to visit Monrovia on my way home for furlough from Ethiopia in April of 1996. I was still praying about where to serve next after furlough, and Liberia was on my short list of choices.

I proposed to join the church-planting missionaries and do some community health type of work around Monrovia after my furlough. I never had to make that decision because soon after I left, fighting resumed in Monrovia. Almost all SIM missionaries were evacuated. God made it clear to me that a return was not His will. I finally left all thoughts of returning to Liberia and moved on to a new assignment in Ghana.

After seven years of terrible suffering and no government, an election was held in Liberia and, like it or not, Charles Taylor was elected president of Liberia in 1997. Really! I heard that people were saying about him, "You broke it, now you fix it." There was some relief from bloodshed but little improvement in the standard of living. Twice SIM tried to rebuild ELWA radio station and it was destroyed. Many of the educated left Liberia. This is called a "Brain Drain," and it was hard to rebuild without those who had left.

It was not just Liberia that suffered. Taylor partnered up with a rebel leader in Sierra Leone, and together they created havoc there as well. In June 2003, the Special Court of Sierra Leone indicted Charles Taylor for creating and supporting the civil war there. Taylor appeared on Liberia national television on August 10, 2003, and announced his resignation as president. He turned over the presidency to his vice, Moses Blah. Taylor went into exile in Nigeria. He was eventually captured at the border of Cameroon trying to flee Nigeria. He was taken to the International Criminal Court at The Hague in Holland. After years of court proceedings, Taylor was found guilty of war crimes and crimes against humanity. He currently serves a jail term of fifty years. I followed this story with some personal interest.

The tribal and economic civil war in Liberia lasted fourteen years, including the years Taylor was president. The infrastructure was completely ruined. There was no running water or electricity in most of the country for over twenty years. Loss of lives was huge. In 2005, Ellen Johnson-Sirleaf was elected president of Liberia. She served a second term. She is the first woman to be president of an African country. I remember hearing of her before the war. She has a degree from Harvard University. Jon Shea's warning before the war has stuck with me down through the years in Africa: "Remain neutral and don't even harbor thoughts of who should govern a country that is not my own."

## THE EBOLA OUTBREAK

The civil war in Liberia was bad enough, but an even worse or as devastating event to the country was the Ebola virus outbreak in 2014. I quote from *SIM Global,* Fall 2014 issue, "As the worst Ebola virus outbreak in history unleashed on West Africa, our ELWA Hospital in Liberia was caught in a sudden and fierce storm. Operating at maximum capacity, staff and volunteers put God's love into action for the sick even as the virus gained ground in the region. Since the outbreak began in early 2014, more than 10,141 cases of Ebola have been confirmed. More than 4,922 people have died as of this writing. And the numbers keep climbing." The reservoir for the virus is thought to be fruit bats. Viral diseases have no cure, for the most part. But with early detection and supportive care, people can survive.

The epidemic dominated headlines for months in the U.S. On June 12, 2014, the first Ebola patient came to ELWA hospital. The hospital staff was ready for an Ebola patient. Dr. Debbie Eisenhut, an American surgeon, and Dr. Jerry Brown, a Liberian doctor, had prepared the hospital to receive infected patients even before the virus spread to the capital. They had researched Ebola, devised methods of how to treat patients, and designed the best protection practices for health-care workers. Dr. Brown helped to convert the hospital's chapel into an Ebola treatment facility, which turned out to be the only treatment facility in Liberia for over a month.

In July, Nancy Writebol, a SIM missionary, contracted the virus at ELWA Hospital while helping disinfect medical personnel during the outbreak. At the same time Dr. Kent Brantley, a Samaritan Purse missionary doctor on loan to ELWA, woke up one morning "feeling under the weather" after working for weeks treating Ebola-infected patients. He recognized the symptoms and went into isolation himself at his home and everyone prayed. He was critically ill when SIM USA office got the call that he would be evacuated to Emory Hospital in Atlanta by Samaritans Purse. He had a miraculous recovery as God used supportive care, experimental drugs, and doctors to help his body fight the virus. Soon Nancy Writebol was evacuated by SIM and she also recovered at Emory Hospital in Atlanta.

In early August, 2014, Dr. Rick Sacra returned to ELWA hospital to provide general medical support in the hospital itself. He was not working in the Ebola treatment unit. He contracted Ebola while in the maternity ward of the hospital. Rick was flown to the University of Nebraska Medical Center in Omaha, where he underwent treatment and survived. I knew Rick when he was a medical student back in the 80s. He did a short-term time at ELWA hospital and, like all medical students at the time, rotated to Tahn to see CBHC work with Marianne and me. When Rick got sick, Dr. John Frankhauser, a SIM missionary, flew to Monrovia to continue Rick's work at the hospital, caring for all non-Ebola patients. Needless to say, triage for Ebola at the hospital tightened up considerably after Rick got sick.

I received an email from Dr. Paul Hudson and Fiona Hahn at the SIM International office in late August, about the same time Dr. Rick Sacra became sick, relaying a request from Liberia and Guinea for the development of biblically based Ebola community education materials/curriculum. The idea was that these resources would be fully immersed in Biblical truth, and that nonmedical people would be able to use them effectively. Attached was a helpful SIM working group paper on approaches to the critical need of community education materials. I went to work that whole Labor Day weekend. I was working at our county health department and was able to print off official CDC materials about Ebola, which was also helpful for reference. By the grace of God, I soon sent Fiona a draft of my work and she made good suggestions. We edited it. It went out to West Africa SIM countries. I did not get any feedback from it, but God knows what, if any, impact it made somewhere. Issa sent it to his church in Sierra Leone too. If this outbreak had happened before I resigned from the mission, I might have tried to go to Liberia and help with the community awareness part of controlling the outbreak. Samaritans Purse was actively doing community work in Liberia at that time, though. God bless them.

Finally, the WHO and U.S. government became involved in stopping the epidemic. MSF (Doctors Without Borders) took over the treatment of Ebola patients. Why did SIM retreat from directly treating Ebola patients? Good question. The answer is three-part.

1. A huge tent was erected on the ELWA compound by MSF with 250 cots for patients. The CDC set up a lab for quick testing and research on the ELWA compound. It became clear to mission leaders that the level of infrastructure and related funding necessary to fight

this battle was way beyond what we as a mission could do. This facility needed millions of dollars.

2. MSF had decades of experience in handling Ebola outbreaks. It was better for those who were suffering to allow those with the most expertise and sufficient funding to care for them.

3. SIM recognized that health care in Liberia in general was in shambles. Many were dying from preventable non-Ebola causes for lack of health-care options. ELWA hospital began to address this crisis by increasing its capacity to help non-Ebola medical needs.

A simple basic rule of thumb during the epidemic was ABC: Avoid Bodily Contact. The famous Liberian handshake was temporarily avoided. Schools were shut down. Government clinics and hospitals were closed. Most Liberians said this Ebola crises was worse than the civil war! There was no place to be safe or get away from the threat of illness.

Someone at ELWA made up a song about Ebola (Tune: "I've Been Working on the Railroad")

No, you can't come in the ER!
First we take your temp!
No, you can't come in the ER!
Just sit on that chair!
Headache, vomiting, runny stomach;
Too much weakness, pain in tummy;
Pain in muscles, swallow hurts him,
Hiccups and can't breathe!
He wants to vomit; he can't eat;
He went to a funeral; touched the body;
Someone near him has just died;
Maybe he's a case.

SIM's motto is "By Prayer," because we understand that everything we do is in service to God and that any measure of success we see comes only through God's help and blessing. SIM set up a seven-day "Prayer to End Ebola" prayer focus. I joined that group effort from September 29 to October 5, 2014. Every day SIM sent out specific prayer requests to end the Ebola crises. In a nutshell, it went like this:

Day 1   Pray that victims of Ebola will have access to good treatment
Day 2   Pray for protection for health workers
Day 3   Pray that grieving families will know God's comfort
Day 4   Pray for wisdom for pastors serving in communities impacted by Ebola that they would know how to care for the hurting
Day 5   Pray that the decision-makers would mobilize resources quickly and effectively
Day 6   Pray that all involved will experience God's strength and comfort
Day 7   Pray for many to hear truth about Jesus and respond to His love for them

It was a blessing to feel a tiny part of the efforts to stop the crisis, even from my little corner of the world in Hadley, Michigan!

I want to mention the Global Mission Health Conference (GMHC) in November 2014, at Louisville, Kentucky. The focus was on the then-current Ebola epidemic. I will never forget in one session, Dr. Kent Brantley and Dr. Debbie Eisenhut were on stage together recalling the days Kent was isolated and very sick at his house. Debbie had to keep his IV fluids going. I wish I could hear their recollections again. There was a standing ovation by over 3,000 medical personnel in the audience.

At the 2015 GMHC, Dr. Rick Sacra did a session on lessons learned from the epidemic. He invited one Liberian man to give his testimony as an example of the impact this virus could have. He had lost over forty members of his extended family to Ebola. He could not finish his talk for the grief that overwhelmed him. He happened to be working outside Liberia at the time of the crisis. He has a heavy weight of responsibility now trying to meet the family needs of those who survived.

The *National Geographic* July, 2014, issue printed a very good article about Ebola, its history and research being done about its transmission. Also, please read the *TIME* magazine December 22–29, 2014, issue *Person of the Year: the Ebola Fighters* featuring Dr. Jerry Brown on the cover in protective gear. It has a fascinating secular article written before the epidemic was even over. It says that the battle was fought with bleach and prayer. By the end of 2014 the number of reported cases in the epidemic from Liberia, Guinea, and Sierra Leone was 17,834 cases and 6,346 deaths. That was only the reported cases.

On July 20, 2015, Liberia was declared Ebola free. On November 7, 2015, Sierra Leone was declared Ebola free. Guinea was the last to be declared Ebola free.

Much more could be said, but I will close with words from the *SIM Global* magazine, Fall, 2015. Dave and Nancy Writebol are now SIM Liberia directors and say, "We have the opportunity to share Christ in ways we hadn't imagined before. We're excited about the start of an Ebola survivors' clinic, which enables us to minister to a whole new group of people who came as a result of the Ebola crisis. These people have special medical, emotional, spiritual and psychological needs that we're able to serve. We're grateful God has opened this door for us to share the gospel." Dr. Rick Sacra has returned to ELWA and is helping survivors deal with complications from nerve damage and vision problems. Ray Hutchison and others are holding trauma healing workshops that are resulting in amazing stories of forgiveness and emotional healing from both the civil war and Ebola. So much healing is still needed in Liberia, in individual hearts and as a nation.

In 1990 our ELWA compound was bombed, looted, mostly destroyed, in Liberia's civil war.

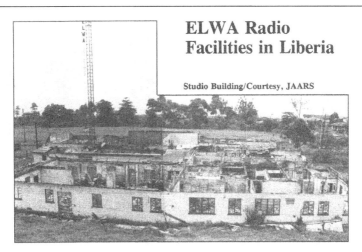

# ELWA Radio
# Facilities in Liberia

Studio Building/Courtesy, JAARS

Inside Transmitter Building/Courtesy, World-Wide Mission

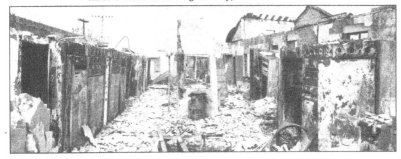

Beach road with felled trees/Courtesy, Carver Mission

Our house/Courtesy, Carver Mission

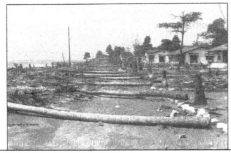
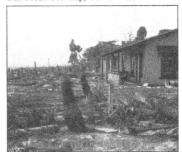

*SIM GLOBAL magazine* article from the Fall 2014 issue about the Ebola outbreak in Liberia.

## THE CALL

Ever been caught in a storm so violent that you wondered how you would make it through? That is what the past 3 months have felt like at SIM.

As the worst Ebola virus outbreak in history unleashed on West Africa, our ELWA Hospital in Liberia was caught in a sudden and fierce storm. Operating at maximum capacity, staff and volunteers put God's love into action for the sick even as the virus gained ground in the region.

**BRUCE JOHNSON**
President SIM USA

Since the outbreak began in early 2014, more than 10,141 cases of Ebola have been confirmed. More than 4,922 people have died as of this writing. And the numbers just keep climbing.

Through it all, God provided shelter in the midst of the storm from the generous outpouring of prayer and support from friends like you. Your prayers were a shield of hope and healing as our friends and peers—missionaries Nancy Writebol, Dr. Kent Brantly, and Dr. Rick Sacra—contracted the disease. Praise God for their healing!

We are grateful for your gifts to help SIM cover the unbudgeted costs of $1 million and counting as we serve the hurting during this crisis.

But the storm continues to rage.

In an interview with Fox News, Nancy Writebol shared that victims who die from Ebola are robbed of their dignity and suffer agonizing pain. She appealed to Christians everywhere to continue in fervent prayer. As you read through the enclosed updates and testimonies (pages 4-6), please continue to keep the people of West Africa, our staff and volunteers in Liberia, and our mission efforts around the world (page 3) in your prayers.

May God bless you for your prayer and support through this difficult time as we serve people in the name of our Lord Jesus Christ.

## ON THE COVER

» With the eyes of the world on West Africa during this crisis, SIM puts God's love and compassion into action by serving Ebola victims and others at the ELWA Hospital in Liberia.

## SNAPSHOTS

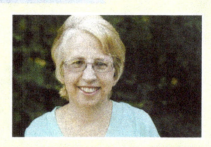

### WE PRAISE GOD FOR HEALING!

SIM missionaries Nancy Writebol and Dr. Rick Sacra and Samaritan's Purse worker Dr. Kent Brantly each contracted the Ebola virus while serving in Liberia. Our SIM family and ministry partners from around the world came together in prayer and support. They were all transported to the United States for further treatment, and have since been released . . . virus free! Thank you for your prayers!

- **Nancy Writebol.** Missionary Nancy Writebol, who tested positive for Ebola in July, was declared free of the virus and continues to share her testimony. She says, "I want to say first, to God be the glory, because he is the one who gives us life and numbers our days. But God uses doctors, and God uses experimental drugs. We don't know whether the drug helped or worked. We don't know whether it was the supportive care, but I'm telling you it was very, very necessary. And we are seeing wonderful results just from supportive care in West Africa."

- **Dr. Kent Brantly.** When Dr. Kent Brantly walked out of Emory University Hospital virus free, he said, "I serve a faithful God who answers prayers. Through the care of the Samaritan's Purse and SIM team in Liberia, the use of an experimental drug, and the experts at Emory University Hospital, God saved my life, a direct answer to thousands and thousands of prayers. Please do not stop praying for the people of Liberia and West Africa, and for an end to this Ebola epidemic."

- **Dr. Rick Sacra.** Dr. Rick Sacra tested free of the Ebola virus and was released from The Nebraska Medical Center Biocontainment Unit where he was treated. "I am so grateful," said Dr. Sacra. "Just so incredibly grateful to have gotten through this illness! Many were praying for me, even people I did not know personally. During the time I was here, there was a growing confidence that God was answering those prayers, and that I was steadily improving. Thanks to God and to the team here at The Nebraska Medical Center!"

# PART THREE

## ASSIGNMENT: ETHIOPIA

### 1993-1996

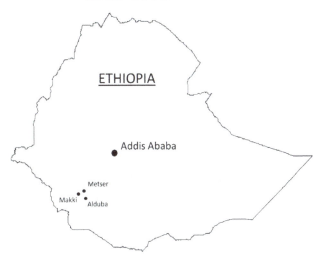

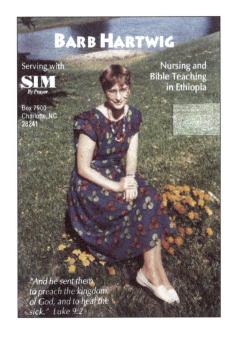

CHAPTER 9

# TEMPORARY ASSIGNMENT AS ETHIOPIA HEALTH COORDINATOR (1993–1994)

*Liberia was still* warring and a hot mess. So when the mission asked me if I would go to Ethiopia for nine months and fill in for their Health Coordinator, Jean Sokvitne, I prayed about it and agreed. I still wanted to return to Liberia, but not while things were so unstable. Little did anyone know it would remain unstable there for fourteen years and that I would stay in Ethiopia for thirty-six months!

I arrived in Addis Ababa, the capital of Ethiopia, at the end of March, 1993. It was about one month before Jean left for furlough. My assignment was to be an office job: coordinator of seven health projects plus the pharmacy stock and missionary health care for over one hundred in-country missionaries. This is, and was, far too much for any one person to do. The administration realized this after I left the position and they split up the responsibilities. It was not an easy assignment at all, and it came on top of the last difficult forty-two-month assignment in Liberia. No wonder I was pretty much drained, physically and mentally, by the time I got back home in April of 1996, only to have the hardest furlough of all. Suffice it to say, most of the 1990s were tough years.

Ethiopia is an old SIM country of ministry. The first SIM missionaries went there in 1927. The SIM- related church was established just before WWII. It was eventually called the Kale Heywet Church (KHC), which in English means Word of Life Church. The Italians invaded Ethiopia in 1935 during WWII and all missionaries had to leave. In spite of persecution, imprisonment, and torture, the church grew by leaps and bounds. When missionaries returned eight years later, KHC had grown from about 100 believers to about 10,000 church members and was running independently from the mission. As opposed to either the church or the mission working one under the other, SIM has worked in parallel with KHC, and I believe this is the best scenario of church/ mission relationships there can be. Eritrea is the one exception I know of where missionaries worked rather smoothly under church leadership. In the 1990s there were an estimated 3,000 KHC churches in Ethiopia with a total membership of about two million. The church is well known for sending out evangelists to neighboring regions. Training church leaders, organizing huge conferences, promoting literature, and radio broadcasts are their main aims. SIM works alongside KHC in their holistic approach to health care and in various levels of Bible training, including youth and women's work. Today KHC sends missionaries to other countries as well, and I got to work with several of them in South Sudan. I say "kudos" to the Ethiopia church, which is truly self-governing, self-sustaining, and self-propagating.

Having resolved back in 1977 at Bembereke Hospital in Benin not to do only health-care work, I looked for an opportunity to teach the Bible. I attended the International Church that met in the chapel on our headquarters compound and saw an opportunity to begin a Sunday School class for girls from grades 7–9. There were about twenty young girls in the class and we had a lot of fun. We learned from one another as we studied the Bible in topics that interested them the most. When I left Addis Ababa for Metser station, I handed the class over to someone else. I still have the nice picture the girls gave me when I left. No one can measure the spiritual impact made in such encounters. All I know is that what is done for eternity is what counts, and the Lord did give us a rapport that was fruitful.

In 1993, SIM had six clinics and one community health project (at Metser) in SW Ethiopia. When Jean left for furlough, it became my responsibility to coordinate them and keep them supplied. Jean was in the process of doing inventory in our pharmacy when I arrived. Helping her gave me good insight into what we had on the shelves and what we needed for the clinics. Each clinic had an agreement with the government, and I was supposed to work on the renewing of one or two while she was away. That proved very difficult, as government officials knew Jean and really did not want to work with me. I was young, could not speak Amharic, and was a new face. It was very frustrating to say the least. Our funding came from donor gifts and a Canadian government source that required a lot of reporting. The fun part of my job was that I got to visit each clinic/station by either helicopter or road. Ethiopia is mountainous and these were rural clinics. There seemed to be endless administrative meetings with field leadership, council, station nurses, etc. Sick missionaries took up a lot of time. I was exhausted every night.

There was a missionary nurse, Sandy Dick, who worked in the missionary clinic half-days to see to routine missionary needs. Somehow, many urgent problems cropped up in the afternoons, evenings, nights, and weekends that I had to handle. I will never forget July 4, 1993. We had an urgent radio message the evening before from Makki station that Maija Carlson, a nurse, thought her husband Jerry had appendicitis. They were the only missionaries on that station. Our field director, Bruce Bond, arranged with the helicopter mission service, Helimission, to take surgeon Barry Hicks (from Australia) and me to Makki the following morning to evaluate Jerry. We were to be equipped to do an emergency appendectomy if necessary. I packed up everything but the kitchen sink. Sterilized instruments, IV fluids, a disposable spinal anesthesia kit, and medicines, etc., were loaded onto the helicopter early the next morning, which happened to be a Sunday. We were thankful for the clear sunny weather for flying and arrived at about 9 a.m.

While I enjoyed a cup of coffee with Maija, Dr. Barry examined Jerry. Barry came out of Jerry's bedroom and said, "It's appendicitis all right and probably not ruptured." If Barry thought it was ruptured, we would have flown Jerry out to a hospital.

Jerry and Maija insisted that we do the surgery right there. We rearranged their living room to put the dining room table near one big window for light. We had one thin mattress on the table. Dan, the pilot, prayed just before Dr. Barry gave the spinal anesthesia. Barry and I had scrubbed for five minutes each at the kitchen sink. Maija was our circle nurse, and Dan held a flashlight until near the end when I saw that Dan was growing faint on us, and I told him to go outside and get some fresh air. Not having scrubbed in to assist in surgery for many years, I was concerned about remembering all the instruments and sterile procedure, but Dr. Barry was very patient and it all went well. The table was too wide, so the patient was on the side closest to the surgeon and I had to lean over the table to do my work. I remember I could hardly stand upright afterwards for quite some time due to the strain on my back.

The surgery took about an hour. My international lesson for the day was that a hemostat in Australia is called an artery clip. We all carefully carried Jerry to his bed afterwards, where he would have to lie flat for thirty-six hours. We had a 12-noon radio contact with Marge in Addis Ababa and were happy to report that we had done the surgery and Jerry was recovering. Maija fixed sandwiches for lunch as we put the house back in order and packed up our supplies. Dan flew us home via another station to refuel, and as soon as we landed at the airport in Addis it started to rain. Surely the Lord was with us every minute that day. Little did I dream that one day I would be assigned to that very station, Makki station, and work with the Carlsons.

I received a letter of thanks written by Jerry on July 23. He wrote,

*Dear Barb, Greetings from Makki. I just want to let you know that I have recovered completely without any complications. The news of the events that took place on July 4 has spread throughout Mursi and Aari country. Now all the Mursi will be wanting such an operation to cure all their medical problems. It was such a busy morning that you probably didn't have time to take any pictures. Enclosed please find a photo. Thanks again for all the hectic preparations you had to make and for all your tender loving care. Sincerely yours, Jerry*

Another highlight of 1993 was our once-a-month Ethiopia Prayer Day when everyone dropped their work and came together for prayers and lunch. We had an hour of prayer for our different stations, an hour for international requests from the mission, an update hour from the director, and some time for personal requests. Those were good times together. Prayer Day was observed monthly across the mission, and I fondly recall our Liberia, Ghana, and South Sudan Prayer Days as well.

Also let me mention the singles group in Addis Ababa that met every Sunday evening. SIM hosted this group, but we had single missionaries from all over the city and many different missions. It was great. John played guitar, and we sang a lot, which was very uplifting to my soul and spirit. We planned many fun trips, and I tried to get away to join in but seldom could unless it was just going out for coffee or a meal at a certain restaurant. One such outing I did get to go on was a road trip up the mountain to an elevation of 15,000 feet, if I remember right. We had a picnic lunch with us. Addis Ababa is on a plateau at 7,000 feet above sea level, which, by the way, means nice weather and no malaria mosquitoes.

Jean returned to Ethiopia in January, 1994. I decided to remain in Ethiopia down country at Metser station where Terry Early (when she was single) had started community health work amongst the Aari people up in the mountains. It would be just Carolyn Ford and me for a few months until Jimmy and Roxanne Cox returned from furlough and went back to Metser. Carolyn was nearing the end of the Aari Bible translation work. There was no mission clinic work at Metser because the local government clinic was established. We had a good rapport with their staff and did community health care in conjunction with them. Before moving down country to Metser, I needed to do three months of full-time Amharic language study. I moved out of Jean's apartment at the headquarters station and down the hall to a little apartment for this brief time. I looked forward to moving down country to pick up the community health work, but first God allowed one very difficult situation to arise soon after I started Amharic language school.

When Jean returned, I never did completely pull away from "the office." As I already mentioned, the job was too much for any one person, and I was helping Jean in the afternoons after language school. I remember it was a Friday about 5 p.m. when our German missionaries from Langano station arrived without notice. Jean and I were still in the office. Herman was practically carrying his wife, Andrea, into our clinic. She was five months pregnant with their fourth child. He said she had had a bad cold and was vomiting.

I could not get a blood pressure at her arm. Our missionary doctor came in to see her. The fetal heart sounds were okay. We got her over to an empty room in our headquarter apartments. I was to stay with her all night. It was awful. She was getting weaker and sicker. She kept asking me, "What are we going to do?" After phone calls with the mission doctor, I finally told him at 3 a.m. that he had to come in and see her. I had a bad feeling about this, and we did not know what was wrong with her. Herman was with their three daughters. I kept nursing notes on her care and around 5 a.m. Jean came to relieve me. They took Andrea to a clinic in the city for an ultrasound of the baby and her abdomen. She was in critical condition.

They decided to admit her to the government hospital across the street from our headquarters where our mission doctor worked. I was supposed to sleep, but around 8 a.m. they asked me to come and help again. Jean was with Andrea and I was to find missionary blood donors. It was field day at Bingham Academy, our mission school. I checked our records and found three missionaries who had the same blood type as Andrea. It took a couple of hours to locate them at the field day and get them over to headquarters. When they arrived, I think it was Larry Dick who took them down to the Red Cross to donate and insisted that the same blood had to be taken to the hospital where Andrea was being treated. Having arranged that, I went over to the hospital. Herman was on his knees crying out to God for his wife. They had started CPR in the operating room.

Andrea died at about 11 a.m. Our mission leaders were down country. Jean stayed with Andrea and could deal with hospital matters in Amharic as I tried to notify leaders. Dick arrived with the donated blood only to find out it was too late.

Herman told his three little girls their mommy had died as they were out swinging on swings at headquarters behind the apartments. Herman insisted we not leave Andrea in the mortuary at the hospital. I called Joe Harding, and he went to the US embassy and obtained permission to keep Andrea there in their cold facility. Jean somehow got her body released from the hospital. Herman called his and her families in Germany and told them. Some of their family members were not Christians and immediately blamed Herman for bringing her to this place. At some point Herman saw her that afternoon and became more upset when he saw that her wedding ring was gone. It turned out she had removed it back at their station. I could not remember if she had it on or not the night before. We were all so glad it was not missing. I had to get a written statement from our mission doctor about her death to send out as official news to SIM and their German mission. I was so upset myself. We all wondered what we should have done differently.

A funeral was planned, and she would be buried at a cemetery in Addis Ababa. Family came from Germany. As to the cause of Andrea's death, she may have had internal bleeding from *placenta previa.* Even as I write this I cannot tell all because of confidentiality constraints, but suffice it to say that Jean and I avoided certain investigations.

For two nights in a row, Herman had a panic attack at bedtime. I was called and gave him a sedative. Then his friend came to stay with him and that helped. I remember going to a staff meeting with mission leaders and telling them that there was nothing more I could do in this situation. I stepped back from it all because I was so upset myself that I could not cope with anyone else's pain. I went over to Brian and Ruth Clark's house to recuperate and sleep and listen to Ruth's wise counsel. Eventually, I went back to language study and we all calmed down and got past it. But I will never forget how devastated I felt when she died. Sometimes I do not understand at all what God is doing. But I will, and I did, trust Him no matter what. This was the second missionary death I was involved with.

On April 30 Carolyn Ford and I drove down to Metser station. I was so happy to be there. I went to Terry's office and figured out what she had been doing in the area. Sound familiar? That's what I did at Tahn when I arrived and Joy Crombie was still on furlough. Carolyn and I lived in a duplex housing unit of prefab materials that had a carport between our houses. Cox's house was empty. I fondly remember the beautiful view of the mountains out my bedroom window where my desk was. This is where I had devotions every morning with Scripture, coffee, and the reminder of God our Creator.

An Ethiopian named Desalyn was our station helper in all things, and he was wonderful. I visited the nearby government clinic across the creek and was building relationships with the community and churches in the area. Carolyn and her two Aari translators were on a strict daily schedule of work. She knew everyone in the area and helped me figure out a lot. Just when I was about to really get moving, I got a radio message from Bruce Bond in Addis Ababa that Jean Sokvitne found out her sister in Canada had terminal cancer and Jean was going home! They needed me in the office again. Oh, no! I didn't want to go, but I had to. Suddenly I was back in Addis Ababa at headquarters. Jean had left even before I got there

I did the office work, but all the while I tried to figure out how to get back to Metser when Jimmy and Roxanne Cox returned from furlough in October. Jean did not know how long she would be gone. I asked Bruce Bond, the director, if I could train Jolene Baker to do the Health Coordinator job and he agreed, and Jolene agreed to learn it!

On November 11 the Coxes and I arrived at Metser. It was wonderful to be back. Carolyn Ford had gone home for furlough. I rode our white mule named Ozzie to a village up the mountain one day and was preparing to do iodine tablet mass distribution in the area to prevent goiters. Jimmy made a helicopter trip to the Bodi tribe, where he had visited many times for evangelism.

Jimmy and Roxanne and I were going full swing into our ministries when the sudden halt came. Only eighteen days after we arrived at Metser, the bad guys came on the evening of November 29, 1994, and we were dodging bullets.

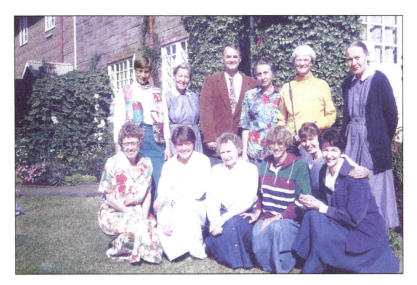

SIM Ethiopia had seven clinics in 1993. These nurses and Dr.
Bascom were some of the staff. We are standing in front of
the SIM guest house in Addis Ababa.
Kneeling: Jean Sokvitne, Jolene Baker, Maija Carlson,
Carolyn Adolph, Claudia, Claire Meckler. Standing: myself,
Lydia, Dr. Bascom, Edith, unknown person, Lydia.

Standing: me, Lydia, Dr. Bascom, Edith, unknown, Lydia

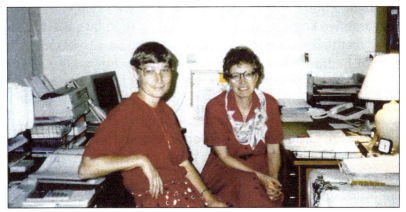

Meet Jean Sokvitne, Health Coordinator for Ethiopia. It was
a lot of work to supervise the clinics and pharmacy, and
meet missionary health-care needs.

## CHAPTER 10

# DODGING BULLETS AT METSER STATION. CLOSE CALL #2

*On November 29,* 1994, at 7 p.m., a direct act of violence occurred against Jimmy, Roxanne, their two boys, aged three and four, and me, who were living at Metser station among the Aari people. I was at Jimmy and Roxanne's house as usual to run our evening radio check-in with all SIM Ethiopia stations. Every day, morning and evening, SIM stations checked in with Marge Scholz in Addis Ababa for business or just a "hello we're fine" report. I was almost finished with the radio schedule that evening when "it" started. Roxanne was washing dishes in the kitchen. Jimmy was in the boys' bedroom reading a bedtime story to them. Suddenly I heard a noise. I thought a light bulb had exploded.

With microphone in hand, I leaned into the doorway, looking for something broken, and asked Roxanne, "What happened?"

She said, "I don't know," and then we heard it again.

This time we knew it was gunfire coming right into the house! I crouched on the floor. Jimmy had handed off the boys to Roxanne. The boys' front bedroom window was shot out, so she had intended to take them to her bedroom, but the shooter was leaning in the broken front window of the living room and pointed his gun at Roxanne. He could have killed her, but for some reason, he didn't. Roxanne hit the siren button beside the front door and moved back into the boys' bedroom, where all three hid under the bunk bed next to the wall for the duration.

Jimmy looked out the window and yelled to me to tell "them" (on the radio) what was happening! I reached up on the dresser from my crouched position on the floor and found the microphone. I told whoever was still on radio that we were being shot at. By the grace of God, Fred at Alduba station was still on the air and said later he could hear the shots. Jimmy dove into the radio room in front of the couch. At least three shots came directly into the radio room. Suddenly, all went still and it was very dark.

Jimmy whispered to me, "Shall I turn on the light?"

I whispered back, "No way, until someone comes to help us; let's just stay down," which is exactly what we did. The shooter did not enter the house nor try to talk to us, but I was petrified thinking he would. Apparently, the loud siren had scared him off. Ever since an armed robbery at the Coxes' house in May of the year before, the mission had employed two night guards to patrol Metser station. When the first shot was fired that night, the guards ran towards the house. From the darkness, a voice shouted to them, "Stay where you are or you will be killed." The two guards ran from the station for help. Desalyn alerted others and one local man who had a trumpet formed from a gourd. A gourd is blown only in times of emergency to alert the area of danger. The man blew it. Finally, national friends from nearby started to arrive. We were surrounded in and out of the house with Aari people carrying their spears and rifles. They had heard the shots, too, as well as our siren and the trumpet.

What a relief when our friends and the local men arrived. I felt very weak and remember just sitting on the floor for a while talking on the radio with our Alduba station and Addis Ababa folks. Jimmy came to the radio and wanted his friend Steve Early, who was in Addis, to come to the radio at headquarters. Steve had lived at Metser with Jimmy before this, and he was very helpful. Fred VanGorkam and company rushed to Metser from Alduba, arriving about 11:30 p.m. They stopped in Jinka, the provincial capital, to report the shooting, so armed police also came to investigate. Thank God for all of them.

We were unhurt, but only by the grace of God. Either the shooter was a bad shot, or he only meant to scare us, or he was only really after Jimmy, or he did not care if he shot us or not. My knees were scraped up from trying to scrunch into the corner of the room. I had peeked round the doorway once early on and saw a man with a turban on his head, holding a long gun. He and his gun were halfway into the front window of the living room beside the front door. We all believe the siren noise cut his visit short. Certainly, it alerted the whole area to an emergency at the mission compound.

The policemen started searching trails in the area for the shooter(s). We could not identify the shooter by face even if the policemen had caught someone. Jimmy said he spoke in a language he had never heard before and had identified his gun as an AK-47. The bad man was not from our local Aari people.

There were bullet holes throughout the house. One went right through the refrigerator freezer and on out the back wall of the house. Each bullet made a lot of holes, so it looked pretty shot up. The very doorway where I first leaned into to ask Roxanne what that noise was, was all shot up. I had been seconds away from being shot in the abdomen or back had I stayed there and not got down on the floor. At about 3 a.m., I decided to go to my house and try to get some rest. Many local people remained on guard all night out in the yard. I lit a votive candle in my own bedroom and went to sleep for a couple of hours. God had spared our lives, and the bad guy would get nowhere near us again that night.

At daybreak the investigation intensified. Shell casings and several bullets were found in the yard and in the house. The police determined that the weapon used was an AK-47 Russian assault rifle. In the morning Roxanne found the Bible story book that Jimmy had been reading to the boys lying open to a picture of an angel standing over two little boys lying on a bed. Shattered glass lay scattered across the top of the page.

We knew we had to leave Metser because the bad guy was still out there. We packed a few things in the morning and prepared to leave. Several hundred people gathered in our yard and Jimmy took the opportunity to talk. He reminded them that no one knows the hour of his death and that today is the day of salvation. He urged everyone to make their hearts right with God. He also told them what their love and concern had meant to them over the last seven years. Jimmy spoke in fluent Amharic language. Roxanne was right when she wrote later that it felt like a funeral as we left. The people embraced us with love, hugs, and tears. We drove our vehicles down the mountain to Jinka, where a Missionary Aviation Fellowship airplane met us and flew us to Addis Ababa. I had only been back at Metser for eighteen days. I had so many plans for community health work, but now I did not know what to do. I was very discouraged. This is one time I should have gone for formal counseling, but I didn't. I called home and told my parents all about it. The day of the shooting, November 29, happened to have been their anniversary. Having another close call to explain was not easy. I don't remember exactly what they said, but I know these scary things were beginning to pile up a bit in all our hearts and minds.

Jimmy was fairly certain he knew what their motive was. It was revenge, not robbery. As I mentioned already, the year before this shooting, Jimmy and Roxanne had had an armed robbery against them at the same Metser house. One of the two robbers was caught. One never was. The Coxes went home on furlough after the robbery in 1993. When they came back to Ethiopia in 1994, they had to testify in court in Jinka that the man caught was, in fact, one of the robbers. Jimmy thinks the shooter was the second robber who was not caught. He may have been out for Jimmy in particular because Jimmy had testified against his partner, but we couldn't prove it. The second robber and the shooter were never caught. This revenge motive theory would come back to haunt me after the armed robbery I had ten years later in Ghana. For now, once again, I would have to figure out what the Lord wanted me to do next. My resolve to trust God, no matter what, was put to the test.

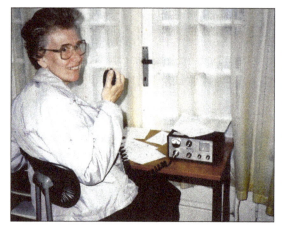

Meet Marge Scholtz, my faithful missionary friend who did the Ethiopia radio schedule to all down-country stations twice a day from Addis Ababa.

This was crucial the evening of the shooting at Metser.

The duplex at Metser station. The open space between Carolyn Ford's house and mine was very handy for kerosene stoves or to wash clothes, etc.

Metser was in the mountains, a beautiful setting.

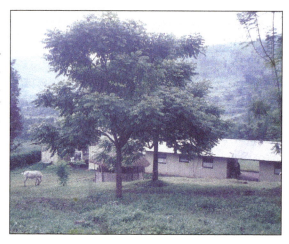

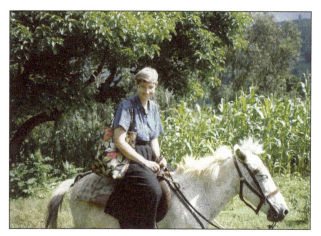

Ready for a trip to villages up the mountain on our white mule named Ozzie. I am wearing culottes.

There are no vehicle roads beyond Metser station.

This is the home of the Aari people.

CHAPTER 11

# A YEAR AT MAKKI WITH THE MURSI PEOPLE (1995–96)

*When we had* to suddenly leave Metser station after the shooting, I was devastated. On November 30, 1994, I was back in Addis Ababa reeling from the shock of it all. Ruth Clark counseled me and was a big help. I remember her saying that the bad guys stole my plans and dreams for work at Metser. We could not return knowing the bad guy(s) was on the loose.

Honestly, I did not want to go back to Addis Ababa, but I insisted on telling my family myself about the shooting, and I could only phone them from the city. The Coxes and I went down to Lake Bishoftu/SIM Retreat Center for a few days to recuperate. Jolene was running the health office very nicely. So when I had a chance to go to the Alduba station and help Sharon Smith, I was glad to leave Addis Ababa and figure things out "down there". I spent two months at Alduba.

Let me explain a bit. Alduba, Metser, and Makki stations were "neighbors" around the town of Jinka in the very SW corner of Ethiopia near the Southern Sudan border. Soon after I arrived at Alduba, Fred VanGorkom (who had come to Metser the night of the shooting) and I drove back to Metser to pack up things and arrange for twenty-four-hour guards on the station until SIM decided on some long-range plans for the work there. I was able to quickly pack up all my belongings and take them to Alduba. There was an empty house at Alduba and I stayed there. I remember that night at Alduba. We returned from Metser at dusk and, surrounded by all my stuff that had been haphazardly thrown into boxes or sacks, I just sat on the floor with a flashlight on, to think and pray. The house had little furniture and it needed a thorough cleaning. It was approaching Christmas. I had no idea what to do next. I sat on the floor that dark night and prayed, "What next, Lord? Shall I go back to Liberia? Shall I go home? Shall I ask the mission for a different country assignment or a different station assignment in Ethiopia?" I didn't know what to do, but I remember telling myself that I didn't deserve nor should I expect to get to do everything I wanted to do. In the Old Testament book of Job, we read that Job said to his wife, "Shall we indeed accept good from God and not accept adversity?" (Job 2:10b).

For the first time in my life, I did not know what to do. The Lord was teaching me that it was not fair to expect no trials or difficulties in life. I decided I would not let it overly cast me down. That was an important decision, given what had happened, and it meant I would just keep on keeping on and trust God to direct me in His time as He always had before. I would keep on trusting God, no matter what.

I worked a bit with Sharon Smith at the Alduba clinic, until one day in December Sharon got a message from home saying her father was very ill and about to have a brain operation. She decided to go home to be with her parents just before Christmas. I was to supervise the clinic, which I did for about a month until Sharon returned.

That was the hardest Christmas I have ever had. Christmas without family is always lonely, but without a home, too, was even harder. Still, I knew that wherever we are, the Lord is there, too, and I tried to get some Christmas spirit. I remember baking a lot. I had stocked up on supplies, expecting to be at Metser for months, so I used them freely. There was one single guy on the Alduba station and the VanGorkom family who received a lot of Christmas baking creations from my kitchen.

Meanwhile, I was in touch with our field leadership about what to do next. Having just been Health Coordinator, I knew what my options were in Ethiopia. I proposed to move down to Makki station and start the immunization program among the Mursi people, which were thought to number only about 5,000 for the entire group. All parties accepted this proposal, and in early February I moved to Makki. There were two couples assigned to this very remote station. The Geddes were home on furlough. I moved into their house and worked with Jerry and Maija Carlson. Maija ran the clinic. Jerry did agriculture-type projects. There were no known believers at all among the Mursi people. They had African traditional beliefs and strong cultural beliefs and practices. The "road" from the town of Jinka to our station at Makki was the worst I had driven yet. The first section of the road from Jinka was known as the Park road. From the Park road, SIM cleared about ten miles of new road to Makki in 1989. It had black-cotton soil that became very muddy and sometimes impass-able when it rained. It was like "Tarzan jungle bush" most of the way there. Our station was across the Makki River in the midst of the Mago Wildlife Park with lions, zebra, antelopes, snakes, monkeys of all sorts, baboons, elephants, etc., all around us. The Mursi people were semi-nomadic cattle herders, and that is why Jonathan Geddes, a vet from Australia, was so popular there. He came with medicine for the cows. Sometimes, the cows seemed to be more important to them than their children. One day while I was out at a mobile clinic, a child was brought to me with pneumonia. He needed an antibiotic. We charged a little bit of money for antibiotics. The father had money rolled up and visible in the hole of his earlobe, but he refused to give any for his child because he said it was for his cow's medicine. I was not sure what to do after arguing with him through an interpreter. Finally, I pointed to his wife's arm band (she had many) and asked for that in exchange for the medicine. He agreed. Many times I took payment in kind for medicine.

Let me describe the Mursi people. The men are usually scantily clothed. They usually carry a gun and their wooden, hand-carved small chair swinging on the end of their gun. Please see the picture of one Mursi man and his gun and chair, with money in his earlobe, eating one of my Russian Teacake cookies. Their cattle are like their bank account. They have to pay in cattle to get a wife and to conduct many transactions between themselves. One day a Mursi man offered Jerry a certain number of cows to take me as his wife. Jerry was going to have a little fun with that, and he actually offered me to the man for 600 cows, which is outrageous, when they usually pay around 30–60 cows. Jerry told me about it, and I was not happy because it gave the false impression that I was available, yet at the same time I smiled, as if there was any real offer there.

There is a spiritual lesson in this cultural practice. What value does God place on each one of us? First Peter 1:17–23 says our worth is not measured in terms of monetary value, but God measured our value by paying the highest price to rescue us from sin through the death of His only Son on the cross.

The Mursi women wear a kind of animal hide that is tanned. They are tall, strong, and do not have many baby delivery problems that we know of. Mursi women have a very distinctive cultural practice for which they are known all over the world. As teenagers, the girls will cut their lower lip and stretch it with a clay plate to form a loop in their lower lip. Supposedly the larger the loop, the more she is worth. One day I saw a woman whose lower lip was so long that it could be put up over her ear. The theory is that long ago the Mursi started doing this so they would not be attractive to outside slave catchers. There is a spiritual lesson here, too. Does God value everyone equally? Yes, there are no distinctions in His eyes. We are all created in God's image and worthy of His love. The worldly prejudices evident in tribalism and racism are so destructive. The wars and offences caused by this heart sickness are huge. Every human being is equal in the eyes of God and when you see the pictures at the end of this chapter you will know why I remind us that God values all of us equally.

Around September and October, the Mursi people grow sorghum to eat because it has a relatively short eleven- or twelve-week growing season. Our station is located along the Makki River, which is low ground and good for crop growing. They keep their cattle up on the plains. Jerry introduced bananas, mangoes, and pineapples to them. He had to hire a guard just to keep the baboons away, though. They are real pests and even a threat to young children left alone. Jerry tried a solar-powered electric fence around his garden, but creatures still managed to get in. The tsetse flies were also pests. Thank God, they did not carry the human form of sleeping sickness. They bite hard and leave a bruise. One must always be on guard and try to brush them away, but by nature they are able to silently land in a place out of sight, like the back of one's legs. Their bite hurts and I had many.

Our SIM clinic opened at Makki in December 1992. Maija ran this clinic, and the people had grown to know and trust the Carlsons. I proposed to start mobile clinics with vaccine for measles, tetanus, diphtheria, whooping cough, and polio. Sometimes, we traveled by helicopter and sometimes by road. Sometimes, we had a good turnout and other times it was all for naught and almost nobody came to our mobile clinic. One day was particularly discouraging because we had gone by helicopter, and the pilot said he would come back to pick us up at 3 p.m. Nobody showed up despite our being told that there were people in that area. What happened was that the day before there had been fighting between the Mursi and a neighboring tribe right where we were sitting. Rumor had it there could be more fighting. We had no way to contact the pilot, so we waited there all day hoping no more fighting would break out. Only one man came to us, and that is how we knew what was going on. Another time, I remember we landed and had crowds of people waiting for us. But the pilot said he would be back at 11 a.m. to pick us up! Oh, no. We worked as fast as we could, but because we didn't have enough time, we left a lot of kids unvaccinated that day. That was very disappointing.

Every month we tried to get to three sites. Sometimes we had a good turn out, but often it was only a few kids. If we went by Land Cruiser, we spent the night in tents. I saw the most gorgeous sunsets ever up on the plains when we camped. I can still visualize this big bright yellow spider on the outside of my tent one evening. This whole experience among the Mursi was not for the squeamish. I was thankful for my farm background, again, which I know helped me handle many things. We called this one tree "Holiday Inn" where we often camped. We started each clinic with devotions when a crowd had gathered. I remember teaching the story of Adam and Eve and their disobedience to God. One of the men asked me what that had to do with them before I got to the application. Good question, and I tried my best to explain that because Adam and Eve sinned, we all have sinned. They heard the gospel message, and we certainly relied on the Holy Spirit to bring understanding to their minds and souls.

The Kale Heywet Church had assigned two Aari evangelists to Makki. The Aari tribe is the one around Metser. One evangelist was named Abraham, and he led the weekly church service at Makki. It was held on the verandah of our clinic. Many Mursi came weekly and listened, including their local leader named Kenamari. If Kenamari ever believed, then many others would follow his lead. No one that we knew of had yet accepted and believed in the Lord Jesus in 1995 while I was there. There were no schools in Mursiland either, so we could not have them read a Bible. The Bible was not translated into their language. Very few Mursi people could even speak Amharic, and so the Amharic Bible translation was not going to be very helpful either. There were so many barriers to the gospel being able to penetrate their hearts and souls. We would be patient and persistent with our witness and earn their trust, and we would show them that we cared for and respected them.

One of the first times we went to "Holiday Inn," the people gathered, but they soon became distracted by some tourist vehicles that had just pulled up a little ways away. Tourists came to the game park and were fascinated by the people, too. They often traded items with them for Mursi souvenirs. That day we went and asked the tourist leader to go to a different area because of our clinic, but they refused. It was the clinic that brought them the crowd, and they were happy about it and did not care one bit about our plans to help the people that day. We waited and hoped to still do our work, but finally we had to leave to get home before dark. That day, I added tourists to the long list of constraints on the Mursi Health program.

One day I was out in the village near our station to invite the local people to the Makki vaccine clinic being held that day. A village man asked me to follow him to one house and see a sick man. I went in and it was Boika! He was a young man who often came to our station and was very friendly. I know Jonathan had witnessed to him often about the Lord Jesus. Boika had been teaching me some Mursi words. Now here he was, almost unconscious! I quickly went back to the clinic and sent out our stretcher with some men to carry him back to the clinic. He had no bowel sounds and by now he was unconscious. I highly suspected he had a bowel obstruction. Jerry and I made the decision that I would drive him out to Arba Minch hospital. It seemed only an operation could save his young life. It had rained, the river was high, and the road would be bad. Jerry put the chains on the Land Cruiser tires. I asked his family to send one person along with us. Our Ethiopian health assistant, Asnake, and I loaded him on the stretcher into the Land Cruiser.

The river was so high that the water came up past the windshield wipers as we kept on crossing, despite the current. Fortunately, the river had a very firm riverbed. We could cross a flooded river with the Land Cruiser because the vehicle's air vent projected up. By the grace of God, we were not carried downriver by the current.

We had left Makki with just enough time to get to Jinka before dark. It was not safe to travel on the roads after dark, so we spent the night there. Unfortunately, our patient was getting worse. At daybreak we took off and went as fast as possible to Arba Minch Hospital. We arrived during their lunch break, so no one was around to receive us. His breathing had been very labored for a couple of hours. He died as we moved him out of the vehicle into the hospital. We were too late. It was sad. His uncle agreed to bury him there that afternoon after I made arrangements with the church in Arba Minch. I only hope he did believe in Jesus and we will meet again in heaven one day.

We did another emergency run to Arba Minch hospital one day with a young pregnant woman whose baby's hand was out. The baby was lying transverse, which is impossible to deliver. I could not be sure if the baby was alive or not. I drove fast in case there was a chance to save the baby. At the hospital they saved the life of the mother, but the baby had died. If we had known the baby was dead, we would not have rushed quite as fast. With a Doppler machine we would have known for sure if we had a live baby. Next time I went on furlough, I obtained a Doppler device, which runs off a nine-volt battery, from the Samaritan's Purse organization and always had it with me in Ghana and South Sudan. It was pretty exciting for a woman and her husband to be able to hear their baby's heartbeat at just four or five months of pregnancy.

After six months at Makki, it was time for the Carlsons to go home on furlough. There was no one else to fill in at the clinic for Maija. I was due for furlough, too, but I agreed to stay at Makki and supervise the clinic until Maija came back. That is how I came to be at Makki for all of 1995 and on into 1996. Thank God for Asnake, an Ethiopian Health Assistant, who saw the patients on a daily basis. I got involved with the difficult cases and did all the reporting and ordering. Maija had taught me how to treat the many tuberculosis (TB) patients we had among the Mursi. Compliance with a whole year of taking medicine for a cure was very difficult to relay to our TB patients. They would get better and then stop taking the medicine. Then they would return when the TB came back and demand medicine again. It was very hard dealing with them because we could not restart them on the same course of medicines they had quit.

Dick and Donna Swart and their three kids came to Makki to fill in for the Carlsons. The Geddes were still on a sixteen-month furlough in Australia, and their house was the family house, so I moved over to the Carlsons' house. It was wonderful working with the Swart family. My diary notes read that in their first ten days at Makki these things happened: we got four inches of rain in three days and another five inches two days later; their dog got tick fever; Donna (a nurse too) put stitches in Dick's foot from a tree accident; we saw a four-foot crocodile in the river where we occasionally swam; I saw a monitor lizard in my yard; we watched a movie on Swart's video player they had brought with them; the Carlsons left by helicopter for six months furlough. In rainy season, this is Tarzan country and creatures come out. Too bad I am not an animal lover to have appreciated all the wild-life! The Swarts thought it was exciting and liked it there very much.

In October of 1995 Metser station reopened with Carolyn Ford and Alex and Theresia Fellow's brave decision to return. After they got settled in, Carolyn asked me to come and visit. She wanted to hear first-hand about the "dodging bullets" event. I drove to Jinka and then on up the mountain to Metser for a weekend. It was good to see everyone there again. Carolyn was close to finishing her Bible translation work in the Aari language, and she was determined to do just that. God did spare them any danger in the months they spent finishing up the translation. The community health work never was restarted at Metser, and the station closed for good when Carolyn left.

I distinctly remember the drive back to Makki from Metser. It started raining as we drove. We had spent too long in Jinka, so we could barely make it back to Makki in daylight, even in the best of times. We should have spent the night in Jinka. I got stuck in the mud on the Park road. We had to use the winch attached to a tree to get unstuck. It was slow going and very difficult driving. For some reason Desalyn from Metser was coming with me all the way to Makki, which was very good. It was very late when we finally pulled up at Makki River. The river was high. It was very dark. I was about exhausted. There was no way I would be able to cross it. Some Mursi men showed up, and we asked them to go tell Dick we were there. Dick came and we shouted across the roaring river about what to do. Dick wanted me to cross it. I did not feel able to attempt it. It was spooky dark with no moon. I shouted that we could just sleep in our Land Cruiser until daylight. I think Dick thought the river would only be higher in the morning, so he waded across the river that night and drove us across! He made it all right, but I still say I could not have driven it. Everybody has some limits and boundaries, and that night I had to say I could not do it. It was risky for Dick to wade across that river, but I could not talk him out of it. Such was life at Makki.

No notes are needed to remember being at Makki for Christmas of 1995. Donna and I had made our big dinner plans, we had gifts to share, and we were going to watch a movie together after dinner. Solar power is wonderful if you can capture enough sun to charge the batteries. Well, at 3 a.m. on Christmas day, Dick and Donna were awakened by strange noises coming from their back verandah. Dick went to check and found that a fifteen-foot python snake was strangling their big dog, Spock! Somehow Dick got that snake off his dog and speared it to death! He tied it to a water pipe on the verandah. I had heard some commotion in the night over at their house, but had no idea what it was until early in the morning when I went over to see what had happened. They showed me the snake. It was still moving a bit. The kids thought it was so cool. I dislike all snakes, to say the least. It had entered their verandah through the little dog door put into the outside verandah door. Their dog seemed okay then, but it did die a month or so later. Dick decided to skin this snake and keep the snake skin as a souvenir. He and Caleb, their son, sharpened their knives and went to work that Christmas morning and skinned it. They staked the skin out on a piece of wood to dry. I will never forget looking out my kitchen window as I was making apple pies for our dinner, just in time to see Dick drag the white carcass of the snake by a rope tied to its head right in front of my window. How unappetizing. Even the Mursi did not want to eat snake meat. It created quite a crowd of onlookers on our station. Jerry and Maija never wanted a fence or wall around the compound. The people were welcome to pass through. Many times they stopped to look in our house windows. This was a good policy, but it meant little privacy, and all our activities were observed unless we were behind curtains.

Something else happened just after Christmas. The Swarts had to take their kids back to school, and I could not, nor did I want to stay at Makki by myself. A nurse by the name of Gloria Millard was visiting from Kenya and came down to Makki to stay with me for a week or so. I was to go to Jinka to pick her up. I had one critical Mursi patient at that time. She was lying in a nearby hut and having terrible spasms in her back. I was giving her valium regularly day and night, but I did not know what was wrong with her. It would be too painful to take her to see the doctor in Jinka, so I decided to consult the doctor. I collected Gloria at the airport in Jinka and we went together to see the doctor. I described my patient's case as best I could in hopes of him telling me what to do for her. Based on my description, he diagnosed local tetanus. I had never heard of that kind of tetanus, which causes spasms in just part of the body. We took medicine back to Makki for her, including the antitoxin shot. When we got to Makki that evening, I was so busy unpacking the Cruiser that I sent Gloria with the medicine to make a house call on our patient before dark came upon us. Gloria treated her and the next day she started improving. Word spread and Gloria was sought after for any and all ailments. It was incredible. The woman with tetanus fully recovered.

That week with Gloria proved to be very important to me because of her experience doing community health work in Kenya with a nomadic people group. Gloria explained how she had trained volunteer men or women in that tribe to do just one thing and do it well. For example, one person knew how to care for eyes. Anyone with an eye problem sought out that trained volunteer. This discussion with Gloria fascinated me, and I began to dream of how I would start up community health work somewhere and train volunteers in just one or two things, so they would specialize their knowledge and skills. The Lord showed me this, and I wanted very much to try out the idea forming in my mind. Little did I know that I would do just that later in Ghana.

The helicopter service, run by Helimission, was very important to us, but we did not want to have to rely solely on it for an emergency. An airstrip had been cleared at Makki. The problem was how to maintain it and cut the grass. Suffice it to say, the Mursi were not very interested in being hired to cut the grass on the runway by hand. Jim Ardill, who was the SIM Ethiopia development coordinator, asked me one day if my dad would convert a brush hog from being run by a tractor power-take-off to being run by a motor and pulled behind our pickup truck to mow the airstrip. Jim was another Liberia displaced missionary on assignment in Ethiopia, and he knew my background. I told Jim that no doubt my dad could do that and I would ask him. Dad agreed wholeheartedly. He and his buddies in Hadley, Michigan, found a good used brush hog and converted it to run by motor. When they had finished making the adaptations, they shipped it out to Addis Ababa by air freight. I happened to be in Addis on a break when it arrived. I can still see his handwriting on the container it was packed in. Hurrah! Now we could maintain our airstrip and use MAF (Missionary Aviation Fellowship) airplanes for transportation. It was always a two-day drive between Addis Ababa and Makki. By air it was only two hours! The brush hog finally arrived at Makki just two days before I was due to leave. I rode in the back of Dick's pickup while he mowed the airstrip for the first time with the brush hog. It worked great, and I thanked God that I got to see it in action before I left! Once again all I could say was "God's time is the best time," a quote often said in Liberia.

I arrived in Addis Ababa for a few days to rest up and say farewell before my flight home via Liberia. The Carlson's were back at Makki. Now that all responsibilities were off my shoulders, I remember feeling totally exhausted. I was tired of all things cross cultural. I was homesick and weary to the bone. I rested and prepared myself for one more thing in Africa before departing for home. I had planned a two-week trip to Liberia in March of 1996. This was meant to help me know where the Lord was leading me for my next assignment in 1997. I had not let go of my desire to return to Liberia.

There is an epilogue to my Mursi story that occurred during my South Sudan days. In 2007, which was about twelve years after I lived in Mursi land, I returned to Addis Ababa for two weeks of vacation. One day I heard that the Land Cruiser from Makki was on its way to Addis with the missionaries and one Mursi man. I wondered who from the Mursi would come all the way to Addis. That evening they arrived, and I was introduced to a young Mursi man named Milisha who was a Christian, spoke English, was dressed in modern clothes, and was learning to read and write in the school that SIM had started at Makki! Wow! God greatly blessed me to be able to meet one Mursi believer this side of heaven. He was the translator at the clinic. Years of work had paid eternal dividends, indeed, as they told me that there were about 200 Mursi believers then.

Please see Milisha's picture and imagine us all meeting one day in heaven!

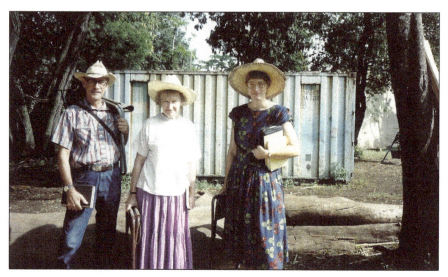

Meet Jerry and Maija Carlson, who pioneered the work among the Mursi people in SW Ethiopia. We are on our way to church, being held on the verandah of the clinic. There were no Mursi believers in 1995 that we knew of.

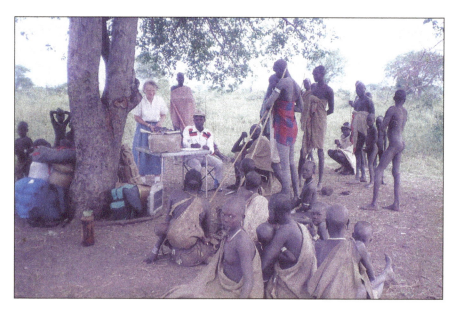

Maija and I are at "Holiday Inn" tree for a vaccination clinic.

See the Mursi women's lower lip and ear lobes that are cut and stretched with a clay plate.

We spent the night here in tents. It is not at Makki, but a couple of hours away where the Mursi graze their cows.

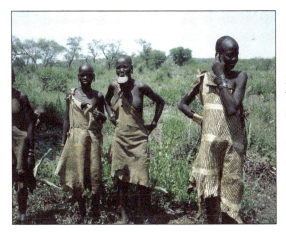

Some young Mursi women. Their clothes are made from animal hides.

Sometimes they melt bullets and make their arm bands.

This young Mursi lady is stretching her lower lip and ear lobes.

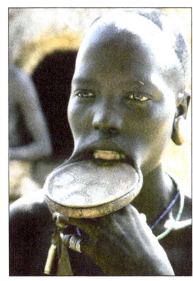

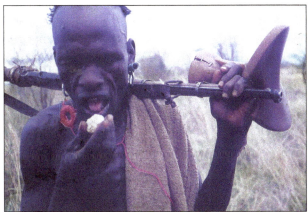

This Mursi man is eating a cookie I gave him. See the rolled-up money in his ear lobe? He carries his gun and small wooden "chair" every- where with him.

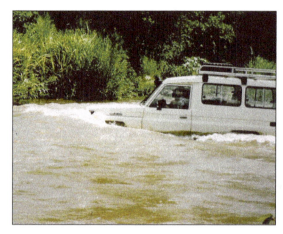

I drove across the Makki River to take a patient to the hospital for emergency surgery.

The Toyota Land Cruiser has an air vent going up, which makes it possible to cross in water over the hood. By the grace of God the current did not carry us downstream. The riverbed is firm.

Caleb Swart and I are putting chains around the tires to get home on this muddy "road" in Mursiland. It rained, so we needed them en route.

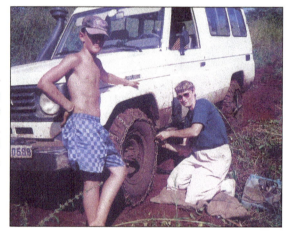

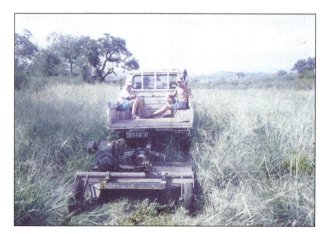

The bush hog that my dad put a motor on, and shipped airfreight to Ethiopia, arrived at Makki just before I left in 1996.

Dick Swart started mowing our Makki airstrip with it for this picture.

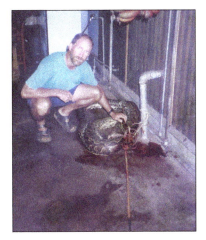

I took this picture on the Swarts' back porch on Christmas day, 1995.

Dick found this fifteen-foot python snake wrapped around their dog at 3:15 a.m.!

Dick speared it to death.

This is the dog that the python tried to kill.

Dick decided to skin the snake and save the hide as a souvenir.

Donna and kids look on.

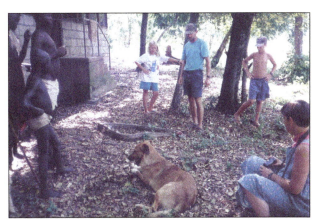

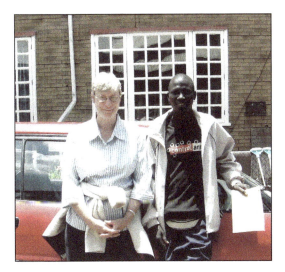

This is Milisha, who I got to meet in Addis Ababa when I was there for vacation from South Sudan assignment in 2007.

Milisha is a believer, can speak English, has western clothes on, and it was my privilege to meet him this side of heaven! There were over 200 Mursi believers by then, compared to no known believers when I was at Makki in 1995.

117

# Part Four

## Assignment: Ghana

### 1997-2005

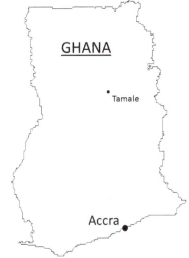

GHANA

· Tamale

Accra ●

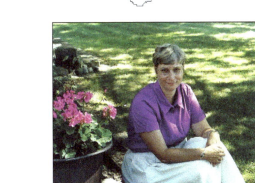

Please pray for
## Barb Hartwig
*Community Health and Bible Teaching in Ghana*

"And he sent them to preach the Kingdom
of God, and to heal the sick." Luke 9:2

with

**SIM** P.O. Box 7900
Serving In Mission   Charlotte, NC 28241

*Assignment: Ghana, W. Africa*

Ghana

## CHAPTER 12

# CHURCH PLANTING AMONG THE DAGOMBA PEOPLE IN GHANA (1997–2005)

*The furlough between* Ethiopia and Ghana proved to be difficult in many ways. When the mission closed Metser station in Ethiopia for good, there really wasn't any other assignment I wanted in Ethiopia. Liberia was still a hot mess in 1996, so I finally gave up the idea of returning there. I was back at home in Hadley, and all summer I had no idea what to do next in Africa. In July of 1996, I received startling news from Ethiopia that there had been a tragic road accident, and our beloved Ruth Clark was in critical condition, paralyzed from the chest down, had fractured ribs, and a ten-inch head laceration. Ruth was with a group in a Land Cruiser going to one station when a heavily loaded coffee truck dodged some pot holes and crashed head first into our missionary vehicle. Ruth was not wearing a seat belt and was in the middle of the back seat. She shot forward right into the windshield.

Suffice it to say, they managed to evacuate her down to a pretty good hospital in Nairobi, Kenya. Unfortunately, they could not do a CAT scan or MRI to determine the exact damage to her spinal cord. She was on a respirator for a while. She needed to return to the U.S. I sent a fax to Brian, her husband, and offered to come to Nairobi and help if they needed me, whether as friend or nurse, and he said I should come. I called our U.S. medical office missionary Dr. Frank Young and asked if the mission wanted me to go officially, or if I should go personally. He said they planned to evacuate Ruth as a stretcher case on a commercial flight and would require a nurse to escort her in flight. SIM paid my round trip ticket.

I had my ticket in hand when word came from Nairobi that Ruth had taken a turn for the worse and was back on a respirator for assisted breathing due to pneumonia. She would not be able to travel by commercial airline after all. I still flew on August 14, not knowing how we would get her home. I had to wait almost twenty-four hours in London for the next leg of my flight to Nairobi, which made this my longest trip ever to Africa. I bought my Kenya visa in the airport at Nairobi, hired a taxi to take me to the SIM guesthouse, and arrived there on day three of what would prove to be only an eight-day trip to Africa.

As soon as I got out of the taxi, Stan Bruning asked me if I was ready to turn around and go right back because the mission had a private medical evacuation plane booked to pick up Ruth. I went right to the hospital to see Brian and Ruth. It had already been almost a month since the accident, which had occurred on July 23. Brian said that he and Karen, their fifth-grade daughter, would go back to Ethiopia to pack up their things and hand over his treasury job. Joy would be a senior at Rift Valley Academy and Ruth "talked" her into staying in Kenya to do twelfth grade and graduate with her class. Of course, Ruth had to write everything down to communicate because she had an endotracheal tube in her mouth and down to her lungs to assist her with breathing. Brian entrusted me to stay with Ruth all the way to the U.S. The med-evacuation plane would arrive on Sunday evening for an early Monday takeoff, and they said there was room for me to accompany her. In the next two days Brian made arrangements, paid the hospital bill, and he and Karen left for Addis Ababa. We were all to meet at Charlotte, North Carolina (SIM headquarters) in a week.

It was not safe to take a taxi in Nairobi after dark, so I spent two nights at the hospital with Ruth. The plane crew arrived on Sunday evening, only to tell us that they had brought a respiratory therapist along, so there would not be room for me to accompany Ruth! I was very disappointed that I could not accompany her too. My commercial return ticket to the U.S. was good, but all seats on that airline were full for the next week. No way would I stay in Nairobi another week. I bought a ticket home on a different airline, and I arrived just after Ruth. It had been a whirlwind eight days of hardly any sleep and jet lag. They did a scan of Ruth's back immediately on arrival, and the news was bad. Her T3 (third thoracic) and T4 (fourth thoracic) vertebrae were smashed beyond human repair, and so was her spinal cord.

On August 21 I arrived in Charlotte to stay with Ruth until Brian and Karen arrived. On the same day I received a phone call from my mother to tell me that my dad had suffered a serious heart attack that day. I needed to go home as soon as possible. My dad passed away to heaven on August 30. He was only sixty-seven years old. This was pretty much unexpected and one sad thing on top of another. Somehow, I got through his funeral, which was very emotional for me. I was exhausted. And I still had no idea what to do next in Africa.

Ken Lloyd called me one day from SIM headquarters and asked me to pray about going to Ghana. I could work with a church-planting team and start up community health work. I needed a stable context in which to work after about seven years of shifting around to different places. This assignment could work for me, and after some discussion with Ghana leadership by telephone, I accepted their invitation to come.

Finally, I had something to get excited about and look forward to. It was going to take some months to obtain a resident visa for Ghana. Then I received a phone call from Elaine Douglas at our mission retirement village in Sebring, Florida, saying she wanted to take a three-month sabbatical and wanted to know if I would fill in for her in the medical office? I agreed to work there until April 15, because it would take a while to get my resident visa in Ghana anyway. It was fun doing home visits with a golf cart around the retirement village and getting to know our retirees and hearing their stories from the time they had spent on the mission field. There was a lot of SIM history to be heard there. I wish I had written more of their stories down like when Zeb Zabriskie told me how he and Bill Naff looked for, and found, land for our SIM Galmi Hospital site in Niger. He said the local chief told him the land was too rocky to be used for farming anyways.

In April, my mother called and said that Grandma had fallen at Riverbend nursing home and hit her head badly. I had just finished my assignment at the SIM retirement village and was visiting at my Aunt Lucy and Uncle Bud's house for a few days near St. Petersburg, Florida. Mom asked if Aunt Lucy and I would come home to Michigan right away and help with Grandma. We packed up and headed home. Mom and the rest of the family were extremely busy with the organizing of the big auction sale of Dad's collections and machinery. Grandma rallied and the auction sale went on as scheduled for April 22, 1997. That was a sad day for me, as I was still processing Dad's death and not ready to see his things go, but it was out of my hands. I was ready to get back to Africa and start my new assignment. This was the only time I did not shed tears when leaving for Africa. My notes say that in my last week in Hadley, besides the auction sale, my Uncle Bob Hartwig had a stroke, a family friend named Shirley Mathes died, and the Ivorys sold their milk herd. Grandma lived until October of 1997 and died peacefully at the age of ninety-seven. She had a tremendously positive influence on my life.

On May 5, 1997, I arrived in Accra, Ghana, West Africa. It is just two countries east of Liberia, also on the Atlantic coast. Accra is the capital city of Ghana, and it is the location of our mission headquarters. I purchased a 1995 double-cab Nissan pickup truck. After shopping, orientation, and lots of business in Accra, it was time to head up north to my new home. I loaded my pickup with all my boxes and followed another family traveling in their truck to the city of Tamale in the Northern Region. It is a ten-hour drive from Accra to Tamale.

I had to live at the Wycliffe guesthouse for three weeks in Tamale while the house that the mission rented for me was being finished. The carpenter was building the kitchen cupboards as I arrived, so I was able to explain to him what I wanted. Finally, I moved in and was very happy to unpack, make curtains, and get to know my new neighbors. Next to me were Pastor Johnson and Lydia Asare and their five kids. We were good neighbors the whole eight years I lived in Ghana. What a relief to feel settled down in a stable country.

All full-time missionaries in Ghana are required to learn a local language before doing anything else. There are five levels of language fluency, and we had to pass level three before anything else. Language learning is ministry because of the relationships developed while practicing it. The Dagbani language was not written in language learning notes. But we were fortunate to have the New Testament printed in Dagbani, and by reading it I eventually learned some more of the language. I hired a young gal named Comfort to be my language helper. She came every morning for two hours and worked with me. We would write a few Dagbani lines to learn, and then in the afternoon, I would go out and practice with some kids, or in the market, or with ladies or neighbors or whoever. My goal became to have a kids Christmas party on my verandah in December and tell the nativity story in Dagbani without notes (see the article about this party when twenty-six kids came to my verandah one Saturday). We had a blast.

I knew a lot of vocabulary and phrases in Dagbani, but the grammar continued to give me trouble. I never fully accomplished the fluency of speaking and hearing Dagbani that I should have. I just do not have the mind to easily pick up another language. I really did try and the people appreciated my effort.

In June of 1998, my full-time language study was put aside by the opportunity to attend a two-month orientation being offered to foreign nurses in Accra who wanted their Ghana nursing license. There were seventeen of us nurses in the group, and I learned a lot about the health system in Ghana. We had two weeks of classes, during which we had lectures about diseases in Ghana, and then we toured some hospitals and even factories. Next we were to do six weeks of practical work, which I was able to arrange to be done at the Tamale government hospital. It was a very profitable orientation time. I received my Ghana nursing license and became more and more anxious to start community health work. The rule was that I could do any health or Bible teaching I wanted to do, but it had to be done in Dagbani language without an interpreter. That was truly motivating me to "get" this language as best and as fast as I could to pass the required level three language test. One thing I would like to pass on about language learning is that it is important to make a certain fluency level your goal. However long it takes to get to that goal is how long you do language study. Instead of saying to someone, "You will do language study for six months," say instead, "You will do language study until you reach level three fluency." One might not seriously study if given only a time frame in which language study is required.

Meanwhile, I was learning about our church-planting work. Mark and Amy Hagerup started it among the Dagomba people a few years before I arrived. Ken and Cora Klay were already at Tamale when I arrived. And Doo-Shik and Gae-Ok Jang from Korea arrived about the same time as me to join the team. Doo-Shik was amazing at learning Dagbani, and he became fluent in the language. He and Gae-Ok are doing well and still serving in Tamale as I write.

We worked in partnership with local pastors and about twenty-two churches had already been started in Dagbon land. These twenty-two churches were part of the Bible Church of Africa (BCA), which is the organization of SIM-related churches in Ghana. The equivalent of BCA is the KHC in Ethiopia and the SIC (Sudan Interior Church) in Sudan.

Crucial to the church work around Tamale was the strategic training of Abukari, Rahman, and Eric at Maranatha Bible College in Accra. They graduated in May of 1998 and started discipling local church leaders. The churches were divided into three zones, and we concentrated on church leadership training by holding monthly two-day training sessions in each district. We managed to raise funds for each of the pastors to have a motorbike. Later, more potential leaders went to Maranatha for Bible training. Having these trained district church leaders was actually the beginning of the end of my time there, because I believed in handing over the church-planting work to nationals as soon as possible.

One of my best national friends at Tamale was Stella. We helped each other. She came over every Saturday morning and hand-washed my laundry and mopped the floors in my house. We usually either cooked or baked something together. She taught me how to cook yams, plantain, cassava, ground nut stew, and greens from the local market. I taught her how to read a recipe and bake breads and desserts. Stella eventually went on to culinary school. Together we put on big dinners for the BCA church leaders at my house for certain occasions, like when Abukari, Rahman and Eric graduated from Bible College. I did a lot of entertaining in Tamale. And I had visitors from my home church during that first term in Ghana. Don Hill and Rich Geigert came for two weeks to see the work. It was a privilege to introduce them all to my friends and local churches.

Comfort was eventually accepted into Tamale Training College, so I lost my best language helper in November of 1997. I struggled on after she left with a few language helpers, but none were as helpful as Comfort. I finally passed my language test later in 1998. I would be going home for furlough in May of 1999, so I did not start training health volunteers before I left. I started to write up my project for approval by the SIM Council in Ghana, talked with local leaders, and began writing a curriculum as well to use when I returned in 2000. Between visitors, conferences, meetings, leadership trainings, etc., I was well versed in Dagbani culture and language, and by then I knew the three church districts very well. It takes a long time to be prepared to make a difference in people's lives. The people need to know and trust you before listening to what you might want to share about a different or better way to live a healthy life. That is the main difference between being a short-term or a long-term missionary.

One day I was leading a church ladies meeting at a nearby village. We had a good group of around thirty ladies that afternoon. Almost all of them could not read, but we memorized a verse from the Bible. Some of them had the Dagbani Bible, and I would underline the verse we were learning in their Bible. It was a nice time of singing, prayers, a Bible lesson with pictures, etc. I happened to be back at that same village a short time later for the well digging program we had going on there. I went to the home of the mother of our church leader to visit. She had cooked food in a covered bowl and offered me some. Before I started to eat, she picked up her Bible and opened it to the verse we had learned together at our recent meeting, and she "read" it before saying a prayer before our meal. She could not read and did not know any English, but she knew the importance of God's Word. I was deeply touched by this evidence that she heard and understood God's Word. She was not trying to impress me. She was leading us to the Lord before eating. It is so hard to measure the impact in our work. Simple moments like this one were encouraging enough to keep on doing the work and let the Holy Spirit speak into people's hearts. For if one was listening, so were others.

My second term in Ghana from 2000 to 2003 was a good one. I returned from furlough ready to start training health volunteers from villages. After much consultation with the District Ministry of Health and our Bible Church of Africa leaders, I went to six villages in the Tolon District and asked them for two men to volunteer as sanitation workers. Please see the next chapter for details on what their responsibilities would be. I spent two weeks training sanitation volunteers in environmental health and clean water.

Next, I went back to the same villages and asked them for two women to volunteer as workers on behalf of pregnant women and care of babies and under-five kids. It was very rewarding to sit with these older ladies and discuss the problems they see among the mothers and discuss ways to improve their health.

I went back to the same six villages and asked them for either two men or women to volunteer to be first aid workers. This proved to be a very popular work. Many sores and injuries were properly cared for before they got infected.

Also during this second term in Ghana, the SIM administration asked me to be the Missionary Health Coordinator for Ghana SIM missionaries. This included giving a lot of advice, purchasing medicines so that there was an ample supply at each station, keeping track of who needed vaccination updates, newcomer orientation, etc. I had done this before in Ethiopia and also at Tahn in Liberia just for our station. I would do it in South Sudan as well. I gave a lot of advice to missionaries about malaria and all the stomach ailments common in Africa. I had good reference books to look up symptoms and treatments for many things. In Ghana we did not have a mission doctor, but relied on national doctors or went to Nalerigu Baptist Hospital in the eastern Northern Region. I think I went there three times with families who delivered their baby at Nalerigu, where they had missionary doctors.

I was at Nalerigu Baptist Hospital on 9–11–2001 when the terrorists flew planes into the towers in New York City. Phil and Andrea Bauman called me that morning and said they were having their baby that day. I drove quickly to the hospital and got there just after baby Cara was delivered by C-section. As I was helping Andrea recover enough to be discharged to the house on the compound that afternoon, Phil was running around doing errands. He kept popping in with news about these attacks taking place in the USA! What? It sounded worse and worse. Meanwhile, he brought their two boys, ages two and four, in to see their new baby sister. When Phil took Kieran, age four, back to the babysitter, who happened to be the doctor's wife, she asked him what he thought of his new baby sister, and he told her, "She's white!" He had never seen a white baby, only lots of black Ghanaian babies. He was not too sure about it all. We really got a chuckle out of that classic MK (missionary kid) response! In the next few days we listened to the BBC radio a lot for updates on the 9–11 crises. Finally, I saw a few pictures of the attack on someone's TV, and my heart and prayers went out to my homeland. It was quite a week!

I had hoped all along that one day another missionary nurse might partner with me in this work. But that never happened. It was too much for one person to train and supervise volunteers in all three church districts. I never could expand into the other two districts as I would have liked. What I could do in the other two districts was work with the government clinics to supervise their traditional birth attendants who had gone through government training. I enjoyed the days I spent with the district midwives and their TBAs. The Ghana government clinics were organized and doing much more than I had seen in rural Liberia or Ethiopia. I had a good rapport with the health workers in all three districts, which is important for sustainability in development work.

In 2001 the Jangs went home to Korea for one year. I was left as the only missionary in Tamale, and the workload truly was too much. The Jangs returned to Tamale just after I left for furlough in 2002. I told the SIM administration even then that I could not do that again. Someone needed to come to Tamale and help me with the church-planting side of the work next time the Jangs were to go on furlough. I hardly had enjoyed a day off for months. Saying that meant setting a boundary, or a limit on what I could do, and I meant it.

What do you suppose is one of the biggest needs felt by a rural African village, especially in the hot dry season? Right, it is water and having enough of it as well as having water that is safe to drink. Almost everywhere one went, the most common sight was women walking with big pots of water on their heads and men with big plastic jugs of water on their bicycles, traveling long distances to fetch water.

I decided to send Andrew Dawuni, a young church leader who happened to be a builder and willing worker, to the SIM water project to the north of us to learn how to dig hand-dug wells. He spent weeks with them and came back ready to give it a try. We selected the village of Kuduo first. After discussions with the village chief and elders, Andrew led the young men of that village to start digging. They dug a five-foot diameter hole down twenty-four feet through some hard clay and hit rock but no water. We found a local contractor with a compressor machine and dynamite. They worked together for six days and went down to forty-two feet and finally struck plenty of water. They were one happy village. Andrew lined the well with curved cement blocks to prevent it from caving in or getting contaminated from surface dirt, yet placed the bricks so as to let the water filter in from the sides. We put a hand pump on it and had a dedication service.

What a job! Andrew was and is a very hard worker. We did this hand-dug well program in several more villages in the next three years. We asked the village to provide the manual labor and pay part of the pump cost, which they willingly agreed to do. This was dry season work only. One wants to go down deep enough to know there will be water in dry season. In the rainy season, we wanted to build latrines because we only want to dig a hole where we know it will be dry in the rainy season. It is not a good idea to dig a latrine hole in the dry season.

I came back to Ghana in January of 2003 to start my third term in Tamale. I should mention that in the week of Easter, 2002, the whole area of Dagbon was rocked by the brutal murder of the Dagbani Paramount Chief and many people living in his big compound about thirty miles outside of Tamale. There was much fear of retaliation on the clan that was accused of doing it. A curfew was still being enforced in Tamale when I came back from furlough. A series of armed robberies had also been occurring in Tamale. There was tension between clans, and all was not well politically, but we could carry on and did not get involved in any of this cultural strife.

Disappointments were mounting in some ways. I was disappointed when a new, single missionary to Ghana chose to work farther north of us. I was hoping to have some help and expand the volunteer training to another district. We had some very disappointing well diggings, too, at a couple of villages due to the type of geology of the earth there. A well-drilling machine tried three different sites at one village at 260 feet deep and still did not find water! Part of the reason there are scarce water sources in some places is due to the ground, not lack of resources. Money cannot get you everything.

Finding qualified church leaders was a huge issue in Ghana. Weak leaders—those who did not learn to read and write, those who disqualified themselves by taking a second wife and so forth—were discouraging. The whole polygamy issue was and is a hot topic that not many pastors want to preach about. In a culture where it is very acceptable, and is seen as a status symbol to have multiple wives, and where having many children is your "insurance" when one is old or needs help, it is a difficult Biblical mandate to have "only" one wife. Many Christians seemed to be taking more than one wife because it "just" meant one could not be a church leader.

Armed robbery became another issue, especially when they came to my house in broad daylight. I have related that whole story in the next chapter. My mother and Aunt Lucy had to cancel their plans to come visit me because my mother had suffered a heart attack. That was hard. My Hadley church was planning to send a group of ten youth and adults to Tamale for two weeks. I really prayed and wondered if they should still come with tensions running high with the armed robberies, the Paramount Chief's murder situation, and the upcoming national election in December, which most said would be contested at best. Well, they did come in August of 2004 and it was hectic, but fun. We were having our annual Kids Camp at the Radach Memorial Center where I was the camp program coordinator. Our Hadley church team helped with crafts, games, and some speaking. It was an excellent time of interaction for them with Ghanaians. Sleeping all ten people at my house, cooking three meals a day, and traveling all over Tamale and out to a village one day took a lot of coordination, but we did it and they all had a good time. No untoward (adverse) events happened by the grace of God. My niece Rachel was among the group who came, and I will forever be grateful for the chance to show her my friends and work in Tamale. She was only thirteen years old. In Ghanaian culture, one's nieces and nephews are considered your own children. Her visit allowed me to introduce her as my daughter (in their eyes) to everyone for two weeks!

In 2004 I did something I had never done before. I went home for my annual vacation. The Ghana election promised to be contested once they announced the results, and that would be in December. I went home for a month, and it was wonderful to spend Christmas with my family and friends. I returned to Tamale in early January, 2005, for what would be my last year in Ghana.

One morning I was eating breakfast as usual while listening to the 7 a.m. BBC news report on shortwave radio. The newscaster announced that South Sudan had just signed a comprehensive peace agreement with North Sudan! Hurrah for the people of Southern Sudan who had been oppressed for decades by the North. Back in the 1940s and '50s, SIM had had a large mission work in Southern Sudan, including a hospital at a place called Doro. The SIM-related church there called themselves Sudan Interior Church (SIC). All missionaries were ordered to leave in 1953. There had been a brief return of a few missionaries in the 1980s, but mostly all SIM missionary work had been halted for decades. Under the new Comprehensive Peace Agreement, the mission would send a newly recruited group of seasoned missionaries to Doro and other former bases.

I immediately felt drawn to this opportunity. I felt that, strategically, the mission in Ghana needed to back off the church-planting work and let the national pastors take full responsibility. Development work will never finish, so I did not consider the community health work as holding me back from another assignment. Also, the mission did not agree to send someone to Tamale to help me when the Jangs went on furlough again for at least a year in 2006. That was a big factor in my decision to transfer to the South Sudan team. The pioneering work ahead sounded fascinating. I contacted the South Sudan director, and he said they wanted to open a training center for community health workers using the nine-month government curriculum.

I was in. God gave me peace about making this transfer to a place much needier than Ghana. The eight years I lived at Tamale, though, were in some ways the easiest assignment I had in Africa. God knows how much we can take, and I needed those stable years of church planting and Community Based Health Care (CBHC) work before the huge challenge of South Sudan.

This would be my fourth country of assignment, and actually somehow I knew it would be my last. I committed to five years (two terms) on the South Sudan team while the Comprehensive Peace Agreement was in place, knowing they would vote for independence in 2011 and I would be on furlough that year. Then I would pray about staying home or returning to Africa.

# Unexpected Challenges... Certain Victory

*by Dotsie Corwin*

This is an article written in SIM's Intercom for the SIM family about Ruth's car accident in Ethiopia.

This article is in the November1996-January 1997 issue.

R uth Clark has always been a listener and an encourager, gifts that led her into a ministry of counseling in Ethiopia, where her husband, Brian, served as mission treasurer. She was traveling to a counseling appointment when an accident occurred on July 23. As she drove with friends through rough country terrain, their Land Cruiser was hit by a truck. Ruth was sitting in the center of the back seat where there was no seatbelt. While others escaped with minor injuries, she was seriously injured.

Ruth was thrown over the front seat, hitting her head where the windshield meets the roof of the vehicle. Then as the truck pushed the Land Cruiser off the road, she was thrown back into the rear seat. She lay there with broken ribs, a punctured lung, blood rushing from head wounds, and her spinal cord severed. She remained at that desolate accident site throughout the night, cared for by SIM personnel, until daylight when an evacuation by air was possible. God's grace sustained her in spite of the injuries and severe pain.

A helicopter from Helimission arrived on the scene the next morning and carefully transported Ruth to Addis Ababa, where an MAF plane took her to a hospital in Nairobi, Kenya. Ruth received excellent medical care until it was decided that she should be evacuated to a large hospital in Charlotte.

Ruth and Brian encouraged their daughter, Joy, to remain in Kenya to complete her senior year at Rift Valley Academy where she is student president. Brian and younger daughter Karen arrived in Charlotte in time for Karen to enter seventh grade in a public school. The family will live in Charlotte, where Brian will continue to use his financial expertise at SIM's headquarters.

The family has many adjustments to make as Ruth learns to live as a paraplegic. As a mission family, let's remember the Clarks in our prayers. Pray for them as they learn to know God in a new and more intimate way through this challenge.

Brian and Ruth Clark, daughters Joy and Karen, and I, before the accident that left Ruth a paraplegic.

We have been good friends ever since I arrived in Liberia in 1983.

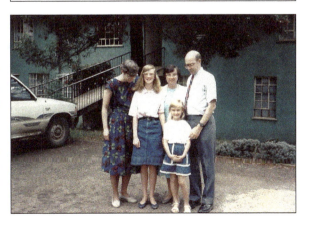

133

# The Dagomba of Ghana

SIM People Group
Profiles

## WHO ARE THEY?

*The Dagomba of Northern Ghana reside mainly around Tamale and Yendi towns. They claim to originate from northern Nigeria. They were warriors with horses. Most chiefs today still have a horse. They are a proud people, but they sense that they are being left behind in an advancing world.*

> Go into all the world and preach the good news...
> Mark 16:15

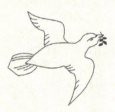

### 1 POPULATION
Estimated to be 448,150.

### 2 LANGUAGE
Dagbani is widely spoken and even taught as a subject in the English-speaking school system.

### 3 LOCATION
Northeast Ghana near the towns of Tamale and Yendi.

### 4 CLIMATE
The dry months, when the Harmattan dust blows in, are from December to May. June to November are the rainy months.

### 5 RELIGION
More than 50% of the Dagomba are Muslim. Some are devout, but many are nominal. About 42% are traditional African religion followers. In the last 5 years God has started to draw these people to Himself.

### Dagomba Culture

The Dagomba speak Dagbani and live in Dagbon territory. They celebrate 5 traditional festivals besides national holidays. After the harvest, beginning in December, many funerals are performed. The person may have been buried for months or even years before his funeral is performed since to afford such a feast is not easy. Polygamy is practiced. They also commonly fosteror rear children of relatives. Jealousy and witchcraft are deeply ingrained in the culture. Diviners, traditional medicine men and land priests carry much authority in health and moral matters.

### Living Conditions

Small villages throughout Dagbon consist of compounds with extended families living inside its wall. A compound has 4-8 rooms in it with the wall around or between the rooms. Grass-roofed rooms are usually rectangular for men and round for each wife. The compound head will have his sons and brothers and their wives and children all living together in a compound. Cooking is mostly done on 3 stones over firewood. Women carry water from long distances. Clean, accessible water is their biggest felt need. Electricity is now reaching into many towns along the main roads.

### Dagomba Government

Two systems of rule coexist. One is government, police and military. The other is tribal cheiftancy who control the land and solve many disputes/crimes. Chiefs are mostly Muslim. The Paramount Chief sits in Yendi.

August 1999

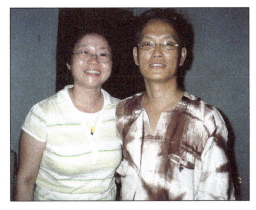

My teammates at Tamale in northern Ghana were Doo-Shik and Gae-Ok Jang from Korea.

Doo-Shik works with the Dagomba church leaders and became fluent in the Dagbani language.

I learned to love Korean food from sharing so many meals with them. They have three children.

As I write in 2017, they are still at Tamale.

Doo-Shik is driving and picking up church leaders along the way for a three-day church leaders training.

We had three church districts and tried to hold monthly training like this in each District.

Those are mattresses tied on top of the truck cab. I taught at many of these meetings too.

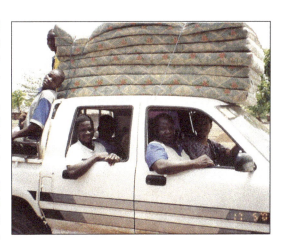

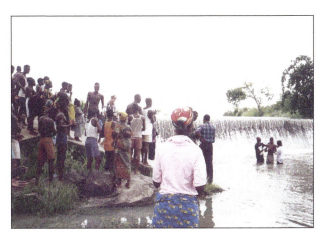

A baptism day. Usually we had to do baptisms in some shallow brown water.

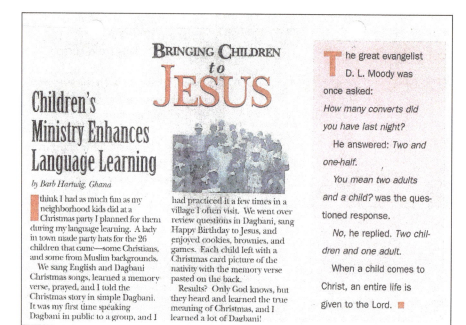

## BRINGING CHILDREN *to* JESUS

### Children's Ministry Enhances Language Learning

*by Barb Hartwig, Ghana*

I think I had as much fun as my neighborhood kids did at a Christmas party I planned for them during my language learning. A lady in town made party hats for the 26 children that came—some Christians, and some from Muslim backgrounds.

We sang English and Dagbani Christmas songs, learned a memory verse, prayed, and I told the Christmas story in simple Dagbani. It was my first time speaking Dagbani in public to a group, and I had practiced it a few times in a village I often visit. We went over review questions in Dagbani, sang Happy Birthday to Jesus, and enjoyed cookies, brownies, and games. Each child left with a Christmas card picture of the nativity with the memory verse pasted on the back.

Results? Only God knows, but they heard and learned the true meaning of Christmas, and I learned a lot of Dagbani!

The great evangelist D. L. Moody was once asked:

*How many converts did you have last night?*

He answered: *Two and one-half.*

*You mean two adults and a child?* was the questioned response.

*No,* he replied. *Two children and one adult.*

When a child comes to Christ, an entire life is given to the Lord. ▪

This is my neighborhood children's Christmas party on my front porch. I told the Christmas story in Dagbani (1997).

The article above is from an SIM Intercom publication.

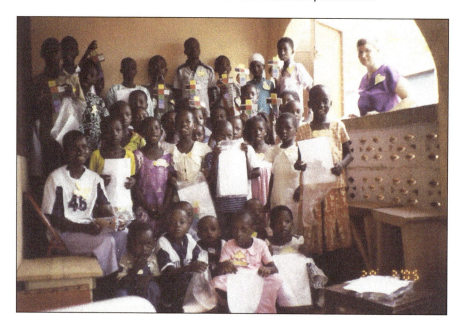

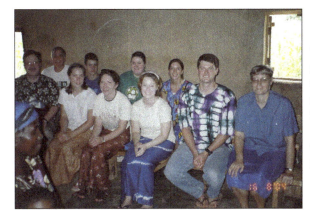

This is the group from my home church, Hadley Community, who visited me at Tamale in August of 2004 for two weeks.

We are sitting at one village church here.

Andrea Bauman when Cara was born at Nalerigu Baptist Hospital in northern Ghana on 9-11-2001!

Big brother Kieran told his babysitter, "She's white!"

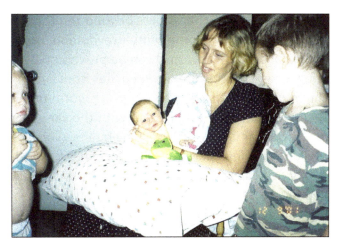

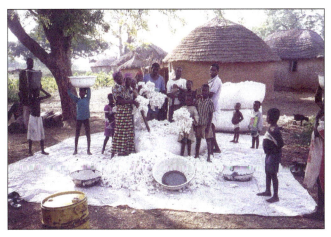

Cotton is grown and sold as a cash crop in Ghana.

## CHAPTER 13

# COMMUNITY-BASED HEALTH CARE (CBHC)

*In 1978 the* World Health Organization held a conference that resulted in a health service called Primary Health Care (PHC). CBHC is that part of PHC that occurs beyond the clinic and hospital. Many clinic patients have community-preventable problems. For example, intestinal parasites (worms) can be prevented by washing hands, covering feces, covering food to keep flies from landing, chamber pots for children, etc. Shall we keep on giving worm medicine over and over again because one is reinfected with the same parasite? Or shall we raise awareness of healthier living habits in order to prevent worms? Africans love injections and pills, but that is not the permanent solution to health problems. On this development principle, I devoted my health work to prevention and promotion of healthier lifestyles on both an individual and village level.

Community-Based Health Care is development work. Development work is different from relief work. Development work addresses the problem of poverty, has the purpose of improving life by raising awareness and mobilizing local people for a solution. Development work is long-term and gradual. Relief work is meant to be done during a crisis when survival is at stake; it has immediate results from external inputs. There is a big difference between relief and development work. I did relief work in the Liberian refugee camp for a while, but I did development work in villages.

### Challenges to Community-Based Health Care

- Fatalism ("but we've always had worms")
- Fears (our ancestors didn't do that)

- "You do it for us" attitude "because we are poor and uneducated" (paternalism)
- Illiteracy among many, for whom new ideas are not so readily accepted
- Animistic beliefs such as "WHO sent the mosquito that brought malaria to my baby" instead of asking "WHAT made my baby sick"

## Principles and Methods of a Facilitator to Motivate Change in Behavior

- Learn the local language.
- Have a continuing dialogue with community leaders, i.e., the chief, elders, head of women.
- Examine traditional beliefs and practices: environment and lifestyle have a lot to do with keeping people healthy.
- Affirm individuals as a person no matter what their beliefs are; holistic health includes body, mind, and soul.
- Transfer responsibility to the community, working with them, not for them.
- Tell stories to get a point across, such as "there was a child in Gondotown with vomiting and diarrhea . . ." which is an indirect method of teaching.
- Use problem-posing pictures for discussion, not solution-posing pictures.
- Use demonstration instead of lecture: for example, literally cook weaning foods.
- Be an example of good health habits; be patient and not easily discouraged.
- Have a solid spiritual base using Scripture as much as possible; for example, Nehemiah was a good development worker.

My assignment in Liberia had been to do village health work and church-planting work, each taking about 50% of my time. When I arrived at Tahn in Liberia in February of 1983, Joy Crombie had already trained village health workers and traditional midwives. I was new and, of course, I did village health work the way Joy did it. In 1984 Joy transferred to another place in Liberia, and Marianne Atzbach and I continued to work that project. It was at the end of my time in Ethiopia at Makki, when I met Gloria Millard, that I had the idea of training volunteers as specialists.

The reason I had been excited to go to Tamale in the Northern Region of Ghana in 1997 was because the mission did not have a Community-Based Health Care (CBHC) program there yet. I would get to start a program from scratch and implement my own ideas. I did it and worked with the local pastors as my partners. I really enjoyed it. I did not have a missionary partner in Ghana. That was fine by me, but I could not expand the program into all three church districts by myself.

In South Sudan, I trained one class of traditional birth attendants. I trained Sudanese students to do CBHC and clinic work, instead of doing CBHC work myself in a number of villages. It was a big decision to stop doing CBHC work myself. Theoretically, I multiplied myself many times over by training others. It required every bit of experience in community health that I had acquired from Liberia, Ethiopia, and Ghana. I had many examples to share with the students of "how to" and "how not to" do community-based health care.

### CONTRAST BETWEEN LIBERIA AND GHANA CBHC

In Liberia we asked each village health committee to give us one man and one woman to be trained in a six-week course as village health workers. We had volunteers from several villages at the same course. We trained all of them in the same subjects, including sanitation, women and children care, and first aid.

When I went to Ghana I asked each village to select two men for sanitation training; two women for promotion and prevention of women's and children's problems; and two men or women for first aid training, thereby specializing all of our volunteers. Sanitation Training and Women & Children Training of volunteers consisted of two-week trainings each. First Aid training was only one week long. We had six villages doing this, where there was either a church or a preaching point. Thus, we specialized each volunteer in one particular health skill. The women did not do sanitation work in the village outside their walled compound in any case, and the men did not do women's and children's health promotion. So why should we train men and women together, in the same course, in everything, as we had in Liberia? We shouldn't.

With the experience of training health workers, I had also trained traditional birth attendants (TBA) or traditional midwives in Liberia, Ghana, and South Sudan. When a TBA went through the training, she was a TTBA (trained traditional birth attendant). These were the grandmothers who volunteered to be on call for home deliveries. In Liberia I attended the two-week TBA training-of-trainers course. It was fascinating, and I came away with a curriculum and teaching aids that would prove vital and adaptable. All of the traditional midwives were illiterate. One must be very careful to teach them on their level. That meant not intimidating them with books or papers, let alone a computer, or even pictures. I taught without notes. Return demonstration proved to be the best way to evaluate what they learned plus, sometimes, I did oral quizzing.

Please see the picture at the end of this chapter of one such teaching aid and let me explain a bit about this. This homemade device is useful to teach about pregnancy and how to space pregnancies. In simple English, the following is how this lesson goes. Every woman has a left and a right ovary (house of the eggs); and a left and right fallopian tube (road for the eggs); a womb (uterus), and the mouth of the womb (cervix). Each month a woman in her reproductive years releases an egg from the house about two weeks from the first day of her last period. That egg will travel down the road for about three to five days to the womb. It is while the egg is on the road that it could be fertilized (I will not be too explicit here). That is what the rhythm method of birth control is about.

Certain hormones are able to tell the house of the egg NOT to release an egg that month. When she stops taking the hormone pills, the house of the egg will start releasing an egg again.

If an intrauterine device (IUD) is in the womb, then the fertilized egg cannot attach to the inside wall of the womb. Therefore, I have never taught about the IUD because it does not prevent pregnancy. I believe that human life begins when the egg is fertilized.

Twins happen when more than one egg is released and fertilized, or one fertilized egg splits in two and produces identical twins. An ectopic pregnancy occurs when the fertilized egg stays on the road and cannot or does not travel on to the womb. Sexually transmitted diseases, such as gonorrhea, if left untreated for some period of time, can cause irreparable damage to the "road," and then the woman's egg cannot get to the womb and she is infertile. Maybe only one road is damaged, or both.

The materials needed to make this simple teaching device are a metal coat hanger bent in such a shape as to be the framework; material packed with cotton are placed on the ends for ovaries; clear stiff plastic for the road with a bead placed to represent an egg on the road; the sleeve of a sweater cut so the wrist opening of the sweater sleeve is the cervix. I have used this device to teach about pregnancy to church groups of men or women or youth; traditional birth attendants; health workers, etc.

Another aspect of CBHC is clean water. In Ghana there was a need for wells in many villages around Tamale. I sent a willing church member named Andrew Dawuni to the Upper East Water Project to learn how to do hand-dug wells. He liked the work. He happened to already be a builder and knew the cement work required to make the curved blocks for lining the walls of a well. The village men volunteered to help dig, bringing up bucket after bucket of dirt via a rope pulley. The last well we dug was fifty-two feet deep if I remember right. We had to use dynamite to blast through mud rock to get down to water. The village helped pay for a pump to put on the well, or else they could use it manually with a bucket to pull up water. That is perhaps the best example of development I can think of: working together with a village to bring in clean water.

Training health workers and TBAs is one thing. Then there were ongoing supervisory meetings with each group. That is a one-day meeting with each trained group every four months. We heard reports of what they were doing and taught them something new or reviewed a lesson; did a Bible talk; ate a meal together; and sold medicines and distributed free supplies.

We always consulted with the local government health department and worked in cooperation with the government clinics. Sometimes they asked us for help. For example, in Ghana, the district health office asked me to assist with their trachoma control program. Trachoma is a contagious eye infection that leads to blindness.

The Ghana district health office also asked me to help with the "Kick Polio Campaign." I spent many days as driver, or gave polio vaccine (just two drops by mouth of the vaccine) myself at an assigned village, or whatever was needed. After several years of polio campaign, Ghana was finally declared polio free! The global Rotary Club helped fund this campaign, and it was an honor to speak one day at the Lapeer, Michigan, Rotary Club meeting, at the invitation of my cousin Greg Potter. I described how the "Kick Polio" campaign was run. They enjoyed the first-hand account of how their funds were helping on the ground.

Interspersed with all these meetings and trainings, I was also treating sick people in villages. I have advised and treated innumerable people for some illness, and I often prayed with them. Praying for and treating sick people has brought many families into the church where they hear about salvation and growing in Christ.

The following is a chart showing the three levels of health care and a synopsis of the curriculums I taught in Liberia, Ghana, and South Sudan.

## CHART OF LEVELS OF HEALTH CARE

|  | **e.g., Fire** | **e.g., Tetanus** |
|---|---|---|
| **Curative level** (hospital) | fire truck puts out a fire | hospitalization where person has a 50% chance of survival |
| **Preventive level** (clinic) | place smoke alarms | give tetanus toxoid vaccine |
| **Promotion level** (community health) | safe wiring | train TBAs in technique of good umbilical cord care |

## LIBERIA VHW (Village Health Worker) CURRICULUM

Following is a short outline of the Liberia Village Health Worker course taught to both men and women volunteers:

    A.  The village health team (volunteer, village health committee, and supervisor/trainer)

    B.  What a village health worker does

C. Good and bad ways to teach people
D. The unhealthy and healthy community
E. How germs move and prevention of sicknesses
F. Safe drinking water
G. Four ways to cover feces
H. Garbage pits
I. Three food groups
J. Child health, including breastfeeding, weaning foods, vaccines, measuring growth, cleanliness
K. Vaccinations
L. The pregnant and nursing mother
M. Child spacing (family planning methods)
N. Parts of the human body and assessing the body
O. Common sicknesses and treatments
P. First aid

## THREE GHANA CURRICULUMS

A. Short outline of the two-week men's sanitation volunteer training in Ghana:
   1. Sicknesses that travel in water
   2. Sicknesses that travel by hands, soil, and flies
   3. Diseases that travel by air
   4. Diseases that travel by insects
   5. AIDS
   6. Killing germs
   7. When to refer
   8. Health without medicines
   9. Reporting

B. Short outline of the Mothers' and Childrens' Health training course with women
   1. About pregnancy
   2. Breast feeding
   3. Family planning methods and child spacing
   4. Newborn to six-months-old baby care
   5. Babies six months to two years old, including weaning foods
   6. Three food groups

7. Measuring child growth and development
8. About immunizations
9. AIDS
10. Fever; coughs; diarrhea and oral rehydration solution and when to refer to clinic
11. Mouth care
12. Reporting

C. Short outline of the first aid volunteer training
1. Care of fresh cuts and scrapes
2. Dirty old wounds
3. Bleeding and nosebleed control
4. Burn first aid
5. Broken bones
6. Animal bites, including snake bite zapper
7. Convulsions
8. Unconscious person care
9. Back pains
10. Prevention of accidents in the home
11. AIDS
12. Reporting

## SOUTH SUDAN CURRICULUM

Outline of the nine-month Community Health Worker Training Course:

A. First Trimester (three months) was nine elements of prevention and promotion of health
1. Immunizations
2. Care of the pregnant woman
3. Malaria prevention
4. HIV prevention
5. Clean water and sanitation
6. Good nutrition/food groups
7. Accident prevention
8. Mass treatment, e.g., vitamin A
9. Prevention of pregnancy/child spacing methods

B. Second Trimester (three months)
1. First aid
2. How to measure vital signs (pulse, respiration, temperature, and blood pressure)
3. Two-week supervised clinical experience to practice vital signs, etc.
4. Anatomy
5. Child health
6. Maternal health
7. Common problems in adults (by system)
8. Introduction to history and physical (head to toe checks)

C. Third Trimester (three months)
1. Do a community development project
2. Six weeks supervised clinical experience
3. Report writing—statistics, inventory, monthly clinic reports
4. Community development oral reports to class
5. Final exams

## TRADITIONAL BIRTH ATTENDANT (TBA) CURRICULUM in 20 lessons

1. Proper hand-washing technique and use of gloves to prevent HIV transmission
2. Female anatomy: house of the egg, the road of the egg, the womb, and the mouth of the womb
3. How a woman gets pregnant
4. Family planning concept and methods (the pill, the injection, rhythm, condoms, and foam)
5. Nine months of fetal development
6. Prenatal checkups
7. When to refer pregnant women to clinic or hospital, or those who should not deliver at home
8. Prenatal checkup practicals with neighboring pregnant women
9. Good food: three food groups
10. Preparation for delivery: your kit of supplies
11. Labor and when to push
12. Birth: cord cutting and placenta demonstration by use of a doll and a square box with a 10-cm hole

13. Return demonstrations by each TBA
14. More on when to refer, including tubal pregnancy recognition and eclampsia recognition
15. The newborn, bathing and cord care
16. Resuscitation of a newborn who is not breathing
17. Normal breastfeeding and complications, including breast abscess
18. Weaning foods
19. Vaccines and well-baby clinic participation
20. Review and oral testing

If you made it to the end of this chapter, it means you have some interest in doing community health work. I never did get to hand over this work to someone else in either Liberia or Ghana or South Sudan. I wish I had. So, by writing this chapter, I hope someone sees the benefit of this approach to address the health needs of people living in poverty, and can see how this work fits in with the work of a church-planting team very nicely. Not many missionaries are committing to this kind of ministry work. I wish more mission leaders would promote CBHC. It seems as though hospitals and clinics are a priority in personnel and available funds. Anybody who knows me knows that I have been aggrieved, or troubled, by this scenario for a long time. I cannot but pass on from the bottom of my heart what I know is a worthwhile long-term ministry opportunity!

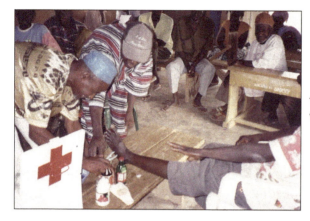

Trained First Aid
Volunteers

Trained Women
Volunteers

Working with
pregnant mothers
and under-five-
year-old children
and babies.

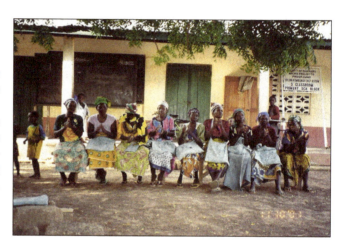

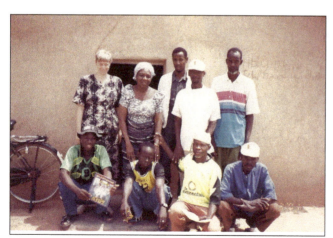

Trained Sanitation
Volunteers

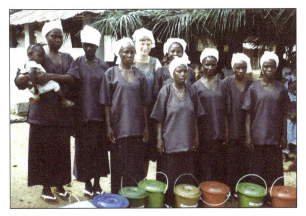

Trained Traditional Birth Attendants. These ladies can do a clean, normal, home delivery of baby. They also learn when not to try a home delivery, but rather refer a mother to the hospital or clinic for a safe delivery. In their bucket are supplies for a clean delivery.

Here I am teaching the midwives how to do a prenatal checkup on a pregnant woman. We invited pregnant women from the community to come to class one day for a checkup. The midwife is going to listen to the baby's heartbeat with a manual fetal scope to her ear.

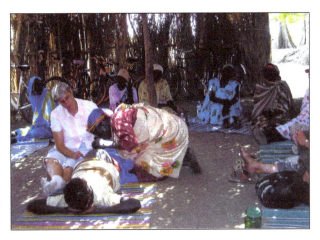

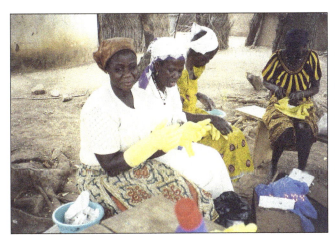

At a supervisory meeting, these traditional midwives are learning to use gloves for deliveries. We resupply them with items as needed at meetings.

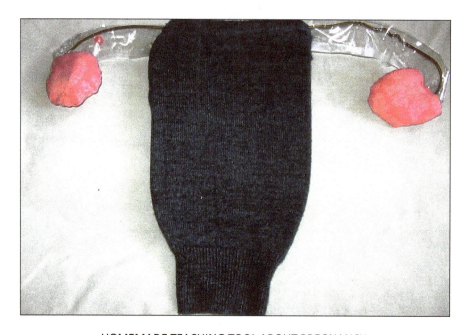

HOMEMADE TEACHING TOOL ABOUT PREGNANCY

The house of the egg (ovaries)

The road for the egg (fallopian tubes)

The egg on the road (see the pink bead)

The womb (uterus)

The mouth of the womb (cervix)

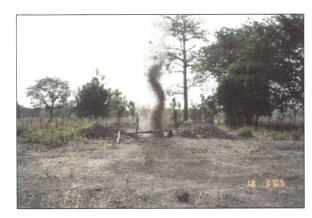

### Step 1

Using dynamite to get deeper in hopes of finding water.

Meet Andrew Dawuni, who was employed by our health project and in charge of the well work.

The pulleys bring up buckets of dirt. Village men volunteer to help.

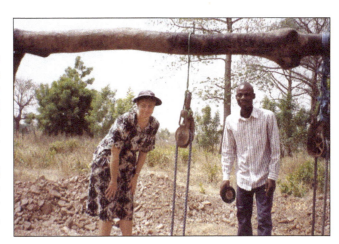

### Step 2

We had this ladder made for the men to get in and out of the hole.

One of our wells was fifty-five feet deep when finished.

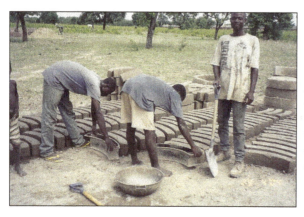

### Step 3

Andrew and crew made curved cement blocks to line the well hole, inside, leaving spaces for the water to filter into the well, of course.

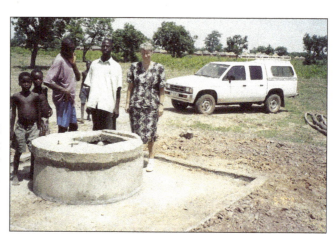

### Step 4

The hole is covered and has a cement apron. Ready for a pump.

### Step 5

This is a locally made rope pump.
Or we bought some Nira pumps.
The village leaders are taught maintenance of the pump and know how to get repairs if needed. It is theirs. They helped make their well and own it.

## CHAPTER 14

# "WE'RE ARMED ROBBERS."
# CLOSE CALL #3

*At 1 p.m.* on Saturday, February 28, 2004, the doorbell rang. I went out to the door at my walled in verandah and did not recognize the two men standing there. I asked them who they were, and they said they had a few questions to ask me. They were well dressed, and one was holding a gray flat file folder. I said they should ask me now, since I did not know them. They said they could not do that, so I opened the door. They sat on my verandah bench with their backs to the road in front. I asked them again who they were, and instead of answering, they started asking me questions, such as when my visitors from the U.S. left. I denied having any visitors and insisted on knowing who they were. The younger guy finally answered that they were from the NBI, which I now know stands for National Bureau of Investigation. They said they came to investigate a cocaine report. I said I knew nothing of the sort and was a missionary. They quickly replied that they knew all about me. They said they had a right to search my house. I asked for their ID. They kind of laughed, and the younger guy reached into his trouser pocket and pulled out a cloth bag. Then he pulled a small pistol out that was cocked open. He clicked it shut, pointed it at my chest, and told me to go in the house and give them all my money.

I hesitated and must have looked confused because the older man then said to me, "We're armed robbers!"

The younger guy grabbed hold of the back of my shirt and pushed me into the house in a hurry. The whole time he had the pistol in one hand and held on to the back of my shirt with his other hand as if he was afraid I would try to make a run for it. I was so shocked. They had fooled me into thinking they were from the government.

Both had excellent English. The older man, who I will now call the "boss," had on a nice long-sleeved striped shirt and dress trousers. The younger man, who I will now call the "mean guy," had on a white golf shirt with a collar, three buttons down the front, and a little red horse emblem. He was very black, good looking, and strong. I did not want to provoke him because he was clearly looking for a reason to hurt me. His pistol was very small, with a brown wooden handle and black barrel. In fact, I wondered at the time if it was even a real gun, but I had to assume it was real and loaded.

In the house, I led them straight to the safe in the storage room and opened it. They kept telling me to hurry and to speak softly. I opened the safe and stepped back. The boss man took out the Ghanaian money in there. It was about 4.2 million cedis, the Ghanian currency, worth around $500 or so. There was a large brown envelope in the safe that held a special offering from the Gumani church. When the boss man lifted it, I told him that it was church money, and my look said, "I dare you to touch it!" He looked inside and pulled out a Bible Church of Africa Gumani envelope that verified what I had just told him. He did not steal that money.

Then they asked me where my money was and demanded I get it quickly. I went down to my bedroom and pointed to the top of my wardrobe. The boss man cleared off a small table and climbed up and found an envelope with $400 USD. It was for a special well pump project at one village. I did not tell them that, or try to stop them. I would gladly give them all monies in the house if only they would just leave.

Then they said to give them more money. I said I had a few more dollars hidden in the hallway. I went to its hiding place and pointed it out. It was about $250 of my personal cash. They wanted more money. I said, "That is all I have, unless you want to get what is in my purse," which I then pointed to. The mean guy became angry. He said, "I will f--- you." I did not outwardly react to him. In fact, I had deliberately been ignoring him and talking with the boss man only. He said it again and then asked me if I knew what that meant. I ignored him. It was a crucial five minutes, because I told the boss man that if I did have any more money I would gladly give it to him. I said, "I'm just a missionary and this is no business office, and that this is the truth." The mean guy then put his hand around my waist and somehow over me. He told me to get to the bedroom and take my clothes off. Meanwhile, I did not comply but looked right at the boss man and kept on talking.

I was being pushed down the hallway now, but I resisted. His intentions were very clear, and with God Almighty on my side, I praise God that he stopped. They spoke in a language I did not know at all. The guardian angels of heaven had intervened, and by God's mercy I was not raped. I was very scared of them.

The boss man wanted my cell phone. I told him I did not have one. The boss man kept opening drawers and looking for more money. He took nothing else. Finally, after he looked in the kitchen, he asked where the bathroom was. I did not want to go back down the hallway towards my bathroom off my bedroom, so I pointed to the guest bathroom across the living room. We moved across the living room, and the boss man saw there was a key in that bathroom door. He told me to enter and I did. He took the thin table cloth off the small table in there and tied it around my mouth. The mean guy came with a rag and tied my hands behind my back. Then they locked the bathroom door and left. Before leaving they said they were not done yet, and I better be quiet for half an hour. I was so relieved to have them leave me alone.

I waited maybe ten or fifteen minutes without hearing any more from them and started yelling out the bathroom window for help. My good neighbors were at home. His daughter heard me yell the first time and ran to tell her father. Johnson came right over. The robbers had left open the door between the house and garage, and they had left my truck door open. They also left the key in the outside of the bathroom door, so Johnson easily opened the door. I had already wriggled the cloth off my mouth, and it was left hanging around my neck. I also managed to get my hands free.

My neighbors, the Asares, were not at home. Doo-Shik and Gae-Ok Jang were also not in town. After I told Johnson what happened, he took me down to the police station, where I told them my story. I went back home and called Ruby, our Ghana field director. Then I went over to my good Wycliffe friends' house and told them what happened. I distinctly remember having an orange soda pop there that tasted so good! Word began to spread quickly around town. Some WEC missionary friends came over and insisted that I spend the night at their house, which I did. Doo-Shik and Gae-OK returned that night to Tamale and we talked on the phone. He came over in the morning when the investigator from BNI came to interview me. He was livid

155

that he had been impersonated. I did not have a daytime guard, and no Ghanaian saw the robbers to describe them. The police did not take fingerprints. They could have and should have, so as to compare any prints with a suspect. All they did was listen to my account of what happened and told me to write it up.

Also on Sunday Pat Robertson came down and stayed with me. I was determined not to leave my home. I told everyone the robbers would not return. They knew I had no more money. That evening, the BNI man returned again to say they were going to do a lineup at the police station in the morning and would I come and try to identify the guys. That scared me. I remembered the Ethiopia shooting, which ended in revenge on Jimmy for identifying one of his robbers. So I declined to do the lineup. Some fellow missionaries were upset with me for that. As it turned out, a policeman later told me that the robbers at my house were not in that lineup, at any rate.

For a month after the robbery, I had visitors almost daily from all our churches. One church leader, Musa, from Zoolanyili, said very sympathetically to me, "If they did it to you, they did it to all of us." What a kind sharing of a bad experience. I received a lot of advice and sympathy from the church and friends. I laughed many times as I related to them that the robbers had to tell me out on the verandah that they were armed robbers. I did concede to have a house guard 24/7 after that. About a month after the robbery, I had a chance to talk with a counselor visiting Tamale. It was helpful. I then went out and burned the clothes that I had been wearing that day of the robbery because they were triggering bad memories. God healed me and protected me from PTSD (post traumatic stress disorder) again. The decision I made with God in 1990 came back to help me. That was to trust God no matter what and trust that He knows what is best and why things happen the way they do.

For some time, I wrestled with God for protecting me a third time from physical harm. Ruth Clark is paralyzed from her car accident in Ethiopia. Is it fair? No. First Corinthians 15:10 says, "But by the grace of God I am what I am, and His grace toward me did not prove vain; but I labored even more than all of them, yet not I, but the grace of God with me." I must not compare what happens to me to someone else in the ministry. I will be and am thankful for the grace of God extended during the robbery.

To summarize, 2004 was a memorable year. It started with the armed robbery in February . In July my home church sent a group of ten to visit me for two weeks. Thirdly, 2004 was election year in Ghana, and trouble was expected in the country in December. For the first time while I was a missionary, I took personal leave and vacation time the month of December and went home. There was some political trouble in Tamale, and I was glad I avoided the stress of all the uncertainties around the election. I had a wonderful time with family and friends and came back in January refreshed.

# Part Five

## Assignment: South Sudan

### 2006 - 2010

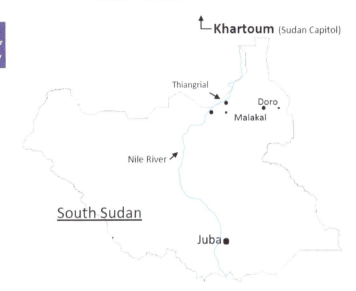

Khartoum (Sudan Capitol)

Thiangrial

Doro

Malakal

Nile River

South Sudan

Juba

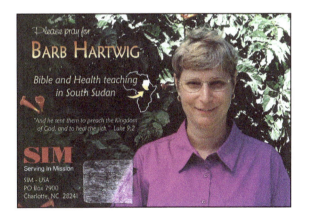

Please pray for

BARB HARTWIG

Bible and Health teaching
in South Sudan

"And he sent them to preach the Kingdom
of God, and to heal the sick." Luke 9:2

SIM
Serving In Mission
SIM - USA
PO Box 7900
Charlotte, NC 28241

SIM
Serving In Mission

CHAPTER 15

# REBUILDING SOUTHERN SUDAN: CHURCH & NATION (2006 AND 2007)

*On January 30,* 2006, I arrived in Nairobi, Kenya, and was the seventh missionary to join the new SIM Southern Sudan team. Our new SIM Sudan headquarters had to be located outside of Southern Sudan, in Nairobi, due to the lack of infrastructure, including banks, roads, and postal service inside Southern Sudan. With the overwhelming task of figuring out how to begin ministry there after twenty-one years of civil war, we went to our South Sudan Church leaders. The SIM-related churches of Sudan call themselves the Sudan Interior Church (SIC), which was founded in the 1940s. SIC leaders gave us five locations to start work at. They said that any training or education ministries were their top priority, even over medical work. We listened and planned accordingly: we would train teachers and health workers.

An initial survey trip was scheduled to each of the five locations. I was to join the group going to Doro in May. Doro is the station where SIM had its medical work in the 1940s and '50s. Jimmy Cox (yes, from Metser station in Ethiopia), Dr. Rob Congdon, Pastor Andrew (a Mabaan pastor from the Doro area), Vicki Beattie, and I were scheduled to fly in a Cessna 208 Caravan airplane flown by an African Inland Mission (AIM) AIR pilot. This felt like pioneer work and I was excited about going! The trip was going to be filled with logistical uncertainties, but at the same time, filled with hopes to be able to commit to an SIM presence again at Doro. Vicki and I became fast friends, like-minded community health nurses that we are. She transferred to South Sudan from work in Zambia and knew Dr. Rob and Nancy Congdon from Zambia days. Likewise, I knew Jimmy and Roxanne Cox from Ethiopia days. We made a good team.

The AIM AIR Cessna plane landed at Liang airstrip. This was my first step on Southern Sudan soil. It was a small, grassy, little-used airstrip out in the boondocks of Mabaan land. I looked around and it was so dry and hot. The pilot was alarmed at the state of the airstrip. Where trees had been removed to clear the strip years ago, there were now sunken depressions in the ground where roots had dried up underground. The pilot said he could not land there again until it was smoothed out because a propeller blade could catch on the ground. When he took off, we were not sure where or when we would see a plane again. Jimmy had a satellite phone for contact. That's all. The airstrip at Doro was a possibility, but was it cleared of unexploded devices? We would have to walk over there and find out.

Meanwhile, the local Mabaan people were quickly crowding around us. Some kids were definitely afraid of white people and did not come close. I knew that look in their eyes. They were curious, but at the same time, hiding behind skirts and bushes. I smiled and was as friendly as I could be reaching out to them. Most did not know English of course. They spoke the local language of Mabaan. It was really good to have Pastor Andrew with us because "everyone" knew him. I couldn't help but notice the effects of the dry season when water is scarce. In many cases people had on ragged, unwashed clothes. I saw a lot of scabies. Scabies is a mite that burrows under the skin and causes severe itching. When scratched a lot, it results in infected, open sores. These are signs of not enough water to wash clothes or bathe frequently.

After almost an hour on the airstrip while we watched the pilot leave with an empty plane, we were led to the village of Liang. It was about a thirty-minute walk. I remember that there were many bright red bugs on the path, which Dr. Rob took pictures of. We had never seen them before. Everything was new and strange, but we were not afraid. Trusting the Lord and knowing this was His way forward gave me inner peace.

We met the Liang village elders and some church people. Pastors Benjamin and Andrew Nita met us there. There was even a clinic building at Liang, but no supplies in it. There was also a church, but it was run down with old grass for walls and roof. To our surprise, there was a brand-new well with a hand pump. Wow! Wonder who put that in and if it was being used yet, considering the signs of scarce water at the airstrip?

In the evening we met with the village people and explained who we were. Jimmy told them we were going to Doro to see what was left there. The church women cooked us a meal. It was their flat-bread made from ground sorghum, called Kissera, and a fish soup. It was good.

Since we had brought our own sleeping bags and tents, we began to set up camp for the night. Dr. Rob did not bring a tent, but hung a mosquito net from a tree to sleep under. Vicki and I had one tent. I remember seeing a bush fire off in one direction. They were burning fields to prepare to plant sorghum and corn crops. It was definitely the end of the dry season. It seemed as though we had just got settled in, when we heard thunder and lightning coming closer and closer. Oh, dear, it was going to rain. Probably pour down rain. It was decided that Vicki and I should move down to the clinic building for the night and Rob would take our tent. It rained very hard and nobody got much sleep.

The next day was Sunday. We were supposed to attend church at Liang. We did not and I don't remember why, but we were accompanied by church folks on a five-hour walk to the county seat, a town called Bunj. About an hour into the walk, we had to cross the Yabus River. We knew ahead of time that we would have to do this. I had put on some long shorts under my skirt. One by one we were accompanied across the wide river. One woman walked with me. The water came up to midchest level and the current was very strong, but at least the bottom of the river was firm sand. No problem. Jimmy gave me a hand up the steep bank on the other side, and I managed to find a bush to get behind and change back into dry clothes (a skirt of course). Off we went again. It was a hot, humid day, and four hours of walking after the river crossing found us at one village just outside of Bunj (our destination). Vicki and I were shown to a room, and we lay down to rest while the guys went into town to see what would be next. Nobody cooked for us, but they kindly brought us "tea." Since we did not know the source of the water and how long it had boiled, Vicki and I did not drink it. We had a hand pump/filter that we used on the trip for our drinking water. The guys finally returned and said we would spend the night there in the village. They had some bread with them, which we hungrily ate. Vicki and I slept with mosquito nets in our room.

Early in the morning, we walked on into the town of Bunj to the County Commissioner's compound. A meeting was arranged to discuss our plans and intentions. It was a long meeting. I remember one leader saying that they knew SIM was serious about returning because they brought two women on this trip. The Commissioner, Mr. Boulis, said that the old SIM compound at Doro was occupied by southern soldiers (SPLA) but had been for only a month or so. Just the month before, they had ousted the northern soldiers and raised the South Sudan flag at Doro. Mr. Boulis assured us that the Southern Sudan SPLA (Sudan People's Liberation Army) were to move out of Doro and into the town of Bunj. SIM was welcome to return. We committed to return by the end of the year (2006). By the grace of God, we did meet that commitment when our Ethiopian missionaries arrived in Doro in December to start the Education Center.

The distance from the town of Bunj to Doro is about two miles. Doro is not a village. It is just an area where SIM had had a big mission compound some forty to fifty years ago. The last time SIMers had been to Doro was in the 1980s for about four years. They were driven away by renewed oppression and fighting from the North. We all walked to Doro on that Monday. The only building standing was the old hospital. It had such thick cement block walls that nothing had knocked it down. One old hospital building was being used as a prison. The other building was used for storage. The captain of the southern soldier contingent had his own grass building to the side, which had been built to be used as his office. This would become our temporary clinic building the following March. We met with the captain and explained our plans to return. He said the SPLA would leave Doro when we returned, which was pretty important to me because I did not want to live among soldiers.

Bricks lay strewn around everywhere at Doro from fallen-down homes and buildings. We hired a man named Nehemiah to be our manager, and he was a faithful, tremendously helpful liaison between us missionaries and the community for many years. We prayed. We walked around and they told us what used to be where. We asked about the airstrip and walked over to it. They all reported that national planes had landed and used it at least twice. They were sure no unexploded devices were on it, and it was in pretty good shape.

Jimmy used the satellite phone and called AIM AIR to report on the Doro airstrip. They agreed to come and pick us up at Doro on Thursday. That was a relief because it would have been a couple of days walking to get to the next airstrip.

We went back to town (Bunj) for the night. We rested at the commissioner's compound on Tuesday, plus we met with just the church leaders. A committee of five people, including Nehemiah, was formed to get a site at Doro ready for missionaries. We were very blessed to have our SIM-related SIC (Sudan Interior Church) people to work with. We depended on them a lot.

On Wednesday we went back to Doro and picked out places for a housing compound and a health worker training center. That would be my work, with Vicki's assistance, until she could get the tuberculosis and leprosy work started. Once the soldiers moved out of Doro and into town, we would clean up and renovate the old hospital buildings for a clinic. It was all very exciting and I could hardly wait to start. The CHW (community health worker) training site would be where a SIM school used to be located about sixty years ago. I remembered talking with Gladys Huyler, who was retired and living at SIM Sebring retirement village in Florida, just a few months earlier about her years of teaching school at Doro. She had kindly told me I should use her house there. It was evident she did not grasp the destruction that had occurred since she had lived at Doro.

I would like to recommend two books written by a SIM missionary to Sudan named Malcolm Forsberg about the early years of SIM establishing the work in Sudan, until 1958 when missionaries were given two weeks to leave. These books are packed with the history and culture of Sudan and the founding of the mission work there in about 1938. They are *Land Beyond the Nile* (copyright 1958) and *Last Days on the Nile* (copyright 1966). I have precious copies of these two books and a personal letter from Malcolm's wife, Enid, who was ninety-five years old when she answered my letter to her in 2007.

We missionaries agreed to live in simple local style huts called *tukuls* to start with, so as to use our project funds to build a clinic, restore the old hospital buildings, and build a new Community Health Worker training compound. Safari tents were set up until one by one some *tukuls* were built on our living compound. There would be no running water, but we could hire someone local to bring water to barrels on the compound via a donkey cart from a community well. At least we had a well for water compared to the other four SIM stations in South Sudan, which had to get water from rivers. We would build a couple of pit latrines. Cooking would be done on charcoal stoves in separate small kitchen *tukuls* around the station. We could buy charcoal in the market at Bunj. Snakes and scorpions were common, so we had to be constantly on alert for them.

Every field had their housing issues. To build *tukuls* we needed to:

- get the right river grass for roofing before dry season ended
- find enough trees to cut for big enough posts
- have a traditional mud/dung floor or a cement floor
- line the grass roof inside the *tukul* with plastic sheets stapled to the wood poles to prevent dirt and creatures from falling down inside
- decide whether to do cement plastering inside over the mud walls, or not
- truck in cement bags and wood from North Sudan markets, entrusting a driver with the cash to pay for it

I had committed to the Southern Sudan Team for five years. Throughout 2006 and 2007 I lived in Nairobi and worked in the new Southern Sudan office while making occasional trips into South Sudan. In 2008, 2009, and 2010 (chapter 17), I would live at Doro and make occasional trips to Nairobi for business and rest. These were the Comprehensive Peace Agreement years in which Southern Sudan was to prepare for independence from Northern Sudan. Due to oppression from the North, the southern people of Sudan wanted to separate from them. The south wanted freedom of religion. Northern Sudan was and is fundamentally Muslim. The complicating factor in all of this was oil, which was discovered in the southern area but bordering the north. Southern Sudan had the oil fields, but Northern Sudan had the means to export and sell it via the Red Sea. Proceeds from the sale of the oil were to be split 50/50. A referendum vote by the people of Southern Sudan for independence was scheduled for 2011 at the end of the Comprehensive Peace Agreement. This was the political context in which we worked.

Soon after I arrived in Nairobi our director asked me to write a safe drinking water project for South Sudan. That was no small thing to research and get approved from our field council before sending the project to SIM USA headquarters for final approval. Jimmy Cox helped with the technical side of the water project, and we came up with a fairly broad proposal of ways to make water safe to drink. It might be wells, or sand filters, or moringa trees, or the New Life water system using chlorine gas.

I knew that the church in Ethiopia was running a large water development program, and I thought it would be useful to see what methods they were using for clean water. So I planned a two-week trip to Addis Ababa for vacation/water project investigation. It was great to be back in Ethiopia and see many of my friends! It was during that vacation that God blessed me to be able to meet Milisha, a young Mursi believer, who I could converse with in English. He told me that the local Mursi "chief" named Kenamari had also believed in the Lord Jesus. I always thought that when Kenamari believed, others would follow his lead.

Another blessing while in Addis Ababa was an evening meal of Ethiopian food with Dick and Donna Swart, with whom I had spent the last six months when I was at Makki in 1995. We reminisced about the famous Christmas Day events around the python snake story. Dick was making windmills to pump water in southern Ethiopia and offered to come to South Sudan someday and see if that would be a viable ministry there. That never happened, but it was a nice offer all the same! It was a wonderful evening together.

One more story about the South Sudan water project. In February 2007 I made a trip by plane, boat, and foot to one of our teacher training bases on the Nile River called Thiangrial to assess the conditions and community resources there for some kind of clean water intervention. I traveled with our Ethiopian teacher, Sisay, who was teaching at Thiangrial. The eight-hour motor boat trip up the Nile River was very memorable. We were traveling northward with the current. The boat was overloaded with people and goods, and I did not move out of the bright sun for the whole trip. I had a hat, but no strings to tie it under my chin, so either I had to hold it on or take it off. It was good to experience the way the people commonly travel because roads are so few. Sisay and I walked the last leg of the journey and arrived just at dusk to quickly set up my tent and get inside because the onslaught of mosquitoes at dusk is such as I had never seen before.

What I found at Thiangrial was startling. There were no wells anywhere within walking distance. No drilling rig had ever been there, the people said, since there is no vehicle road to Thiangrial. The soil is black-cotton clay in which no well hole will find water in, in any case. There is no sand on the shore of the Nile, and there are no stones in the area, either, which means making cement would not be possible without importing sand and stone, too, which ended any thought of trying a hand-dug well. We would have to bring in a water purifier system for the Nile River water that everyone in the area drank. It made sense because their problem was not lack of water, but lack of clean water. I helped Sisay build a latrine while there that week.

The highlight of my week at Thiangrial was an invitation to teach Bible one morning at their village primary school. About thirty kids were in their upper primary school, and I taught them from John, chapter 3. I asked them to write down verse 16, which I had written on the chalkboard. I went around to look at everyone's writing and gave individual attention and encouragement to each student. Their teacher was a student of Sisay in our teacher training Basic Education Learning Center (BELC). I really enjoyed that trip. We ate fresh tilapia fish from the Nile River. By 7:15 every evening the mosquitoes came out in droves! Early to bed (under a mosquito net), early to rise, is wise at Thiangrial on the shore of the Nile.

After this survey trip, Jimmy Cox and I returned by plane in November with a new water treatment system using chlorination. It was from New Life International, which is based in Underwood, Indiana. Using a solar-powered submersible pump, river water was pumped into a tank for sedimentation overnight. In a second tank, all germs in the water are killed when simple solar-powered equipment converts the sodium chloride in common salt water to chlorine gas. The water is then pumped into a third tank and is ready to drink. This clean water was made available to everyone in the village. We held community meetings about the need for clean water and how to maintain the system. I took a microscope with me and looked at a random water sample from the river. Sure enough, something live was moving around on the slide, which everyone was welcome to come and see. By the grace of God, the taste of the purified water was not affected by the chlorine gas, or else the people probably would not have drunk it. Eventually, this water system was set up at two other stations for our missionaries to use.

Throughout 2006 and 2007 the South Sudan team was blessed to welcome new national (African) missionaries from the SIM-related churches in Nigeria and Ethiopia. Sisay was one of them. We helped our new missionaries from Ethiopia and Nigeria with orientation, and they were soon ready to work in Southern Sudan. Jimmy Cox had been traveling to all five stations to check out each situation and to make arrangements for living there. We decided to start a three-year teacher-training, Basic Education Learning Center (BELC) at each of the stations. Our Ethiopian and Nigerian missionaries would be the teachers. They proved to be very adaptable to the culture and rough-living situation in order to get the work started. Each BELC had twenty-five adult students, and I am happy to report that all five BELCs did graduate their students by 2010 (before independence)!

One day I went to our SIM Sudan director, Laiu Fachhai, who was from India, and explained that our new field needed a health coordinator for its missionaries. He agreed, and, of course, he landed me with the job of starting this. I spent considerable time in the office keeping track of everyone's vaccinations, some records, always advising for health needs, and putting together a trunk of medicines, instructions, first aid supplies, etc., for each of our five stations.

Our Ethiopian missionaries arrived to live at Doro by the end of 2006. We barely met our promise to the commissioner to be present by then! By the grace of God, Dr. Rob Congdon persisted in this whole start up on the ground at Doro. He asked the church to come and help build a fence around our housing compound, mostly to keep out animals. At first no one showed up and it was very discouraging. As help arrived from the church, things gradually started to take shape in 2007. It was very sub-standard living for quite a while.

We had a difficult year throughout 2007 at all five new stations. Supplies within Southern Sudan were very limited. We had to hire truck drivers to go to markets in North Sudan to buy building materials. I was in and out of Doro with building teams several times in 2007. The CHW (community health worker) school building cement foundation was started by Ray and Anne Lee. Word reached us that the partially finished roofing had blown down in a bad storm. Our hired Kenyan builder, John Maruti, was sent out to work full time and finish the classroom/office building. Ready or not, I was going to start training on January 28, 2008.

There was one evening in November, 2007, at Doro that no one who was there could ever forget. Dr. Rob had organized a Mabaan SIC church conference in Bunj with a speaker from Zambia named Pastor John. Rod and Mike, short-term builders, were there. John Maruti was also there, and Vicki and I. I was the cook for everyone. As we were just finishing praying together one night after supper in the dining room, someone ran up in the dark yelling "snake, snake" in Arabic. John jumped up and others followed. The guard was alerted to it by our station cat, if I remember right. It was a huge snake, and it had gone down between Vicki's *tukul* and the latrine. Dr. Rob had very swollen, red eyes from conjunctivitis, so he could not see well, but he went out to search anyway. John had just grabbed a big piece of wood and he spotted the snake. It was a seven-foot Egyptian cobra (deadly)! John wounded it, but it slithered away. Joseph, the watchman, kept on looking for it, and twenty minutes later hollered that he found it. Of course, I was staying back just watching when four men came up to me out of the dark, soldiers, smelling of alcohol and tobacco, and demanded the doctor see a sick baby they had with them immediately. I explained about the snake search, but they would not wait and demanded to see Dr. Rob. I called Rob and he saw their newborn baby, who indeed was very sick. Dr. Rob and Amy started an IV, but we did not have the right antibiotic and the baby died. Meanwhile, John and Joseph did kill the big snake. What an evening. It was midnight before we all settled down for the night.

I sent out a letter to SIC churches asking them to recommend adults with at least a seventh-grade education to apply for CHW training. Most of our students went to school in the refugee camps of Ethiopia. Vicki and I interviewed many applicants and selected twelve from among them for our first class of 2008. Part of the entrance test and interview were a couple of simple story problems. One story problem was that a teacher had five students. The teacher was given twenty mangoes for the students. How many mangoes would he give to each student? This is a division test, right? Well, this applicant said he would only give three mangoes to each student. He would not give out all the mangoes at one time. No way. He answered with his culture background and would not just do the division. We ended up accepting him as one of our twelve students, but we shouldn't have. He was difficult and would not do the required work, so finally Vicki had to expel him from the school.

Our first class of twelve students were selected, the new classroom/office building was coming along, and we had told each student to arrive on January 28, 2008. Vicki and I needed some time to sit down and make lesson plans. God gave us a week to do that uninterrupted in Nairobi when the Kenya election on December 27, 2007, ended with trouble in the streets, and everyone was house-bound while the government of Kenya settled the results of their election. It was the perfect time for us to make daily lesson plans for the first trimester based on the Sudan curriculum objectives we had. Vicki and I had a rented apartment in Nairobi and really enjoyed these preparation days. It was a nice distraction from the serious trouble going on outside!

I knew I would go on furlough in May of 2008, and I wanted to see everything going smoothly by the time I left Vicki to complete the year with our first class of students. We were highly disappointed when the experienced, short-term nurse we thought was coming to replace me was not accepted by SIM. What a blow. Now what? No one could do this training alone, as it was the first year of the course. Dr. Masters was going to help Vicki with the school, but he died before that could happen. After I left for furlough, they found a nurse to assist Vicki, but it was rough for them and the students until graduation time in November. Perhaps, with hindsight, we should have sent the students home after the first trimester when I left, and had them return in January 2009, to finish the course when I returned.

Vicki had already moved to Doro in April 2007 and had a *tukul*, but I moved to Doro in early January of 2008. My *tukul* was gradually being built, so I would have to live in a safari tent on the mission compound. It had no shade. It was so hot inside my tent. I just wilted and sweated and spent as little time as possible in there. We had a dining hall, and I preferred to be in there or at the school office working or in our little kitchen *tukul* that was right beside my tent.

The first four months of living at Doro were difficult days in the heat of the dry season, with a new program to teach, making sure the students were fed three meals a day, leadership team responsibilities on the station, cooking, entertaining visitors and work groups, plus UN meetings about the repatriation of Southern Sudanese from Ethiopia refugee camps to Doro. Somehow Vicki and I also began teaching TBAs in Bunj one morning a week. I was more than ready for furlough in May. I was weary of everything and needed a break. Even if Vicki had to close the school until I returned, I really needed to take a break. Oh, I would be back without question in January 2009, but two and a half years were enough and I was going home. My niece Rachel, who visited me at Tamale in Ghana, was graduating from high school the third weekend of May and I promised to be there.

I packed up, said farewells, and was headed for furlough when the plane crashed at Doro on takeoff. "Lord, sometimes I don't get it. I gave this all I had and am about exhausted. But You say the challenges are not over yet. Yes, Lord, I do trust You, no matter what." Good thing I made that firm decision back in 1990. R. A. Torrey said it like this: "The reason why many fail in battle is because they wait until the hour of battle. The reason why others succeed in battle is because they have gained their victory on their knees long before the battle came. . . Anticipate your battles; fight them on your knees before temptation comes, and you will always have victory."

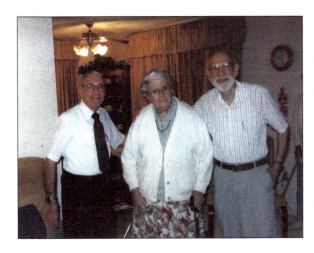

I must give tribute to these retired Sudan missionaries, Mr. Bill Rogers, Miss Gladys Huyler, and Mr. Chuck Guth. They were at Doro in the 1940s and early '50s. I met them at our SIM retirement village in Sebring, Florida.

Dr. Dave Bremner was the speaker at our first Sudan Spiritual Life Conference. One of my office jobs in 2007 was to coordinate the program for this conference. We were a good team and very international.

**SIM** PROJECT NEWS APRIL 2007
REBUILDING SOUTHERN SUDAN: CHURCH & NATION

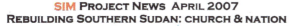

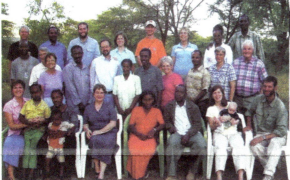

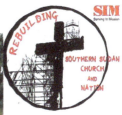

You may have noticed our program is called **Rebuilding Southern Sudan: Church & Nation**. We intentionally listed "Church" first because despite all the good development work we do, our primary focus is still strengthening God's church in Sudan.

*"... the church, you see, is not peripheral to the world, the world is peripheral to the church."* Ephesians 1.22 (the Message)

*It is no small feat getting the Rebuilding team together in one place! We are spread out between our administrative base in Kenya & our project bases in southern Sudan. But recently we met half-way, near the Kenya/Sudan border, for our first ever **Spiritual Life Conference** It was a blessed time for us as we shared ministry reports, studied God's word, prayed, sang and worshipped together. The fellowship was precious! Sadly, our Nigerian missionaries are missing due to visa problems.*

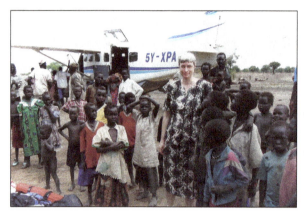

My first step on South Sudan soil in May 2006.

The AIM AIR plane dropped us off at Liang and picked us up at Doro.

We all had to cross the Yabus River en route from Liang to Doro, a five-hour walk.

We were going to Doro to decide whether the time was right to return.

Dr. Rob Congdon, Jimmy Cox, Vicki Beattie, and I made the trip with church leaders.

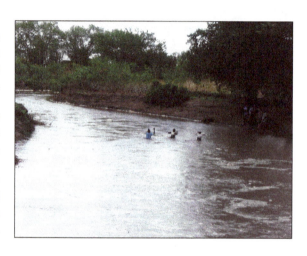

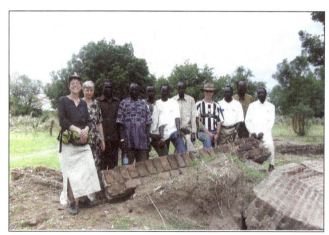

When we got to Doro, we found almost everything destroyed. This used to be a school site, as was explained to us by the church leaders who remembered. Gladys Huyler probably taught here. We decided to build the Health Workers School beside these ruins.

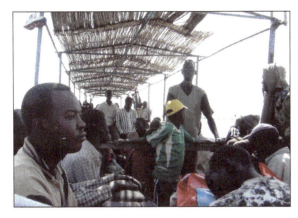

I took this picture of my left-hand view on the Nile River boat. It was an eight-hour trip one day from Malakal to our Thiangrial station.

Sisay, our Ethiopian missionary, was with me. He lived there as the teacher of our Basic Education Learning Center (BELC) in Thiangrial.

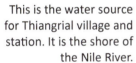

This is the water source for Thiangrial village and station. It is the shore of the Nile River.

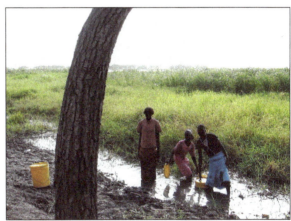

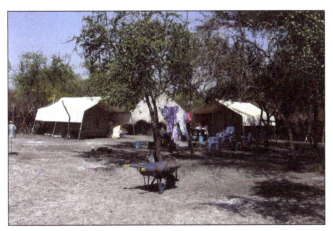

This is our SIM Thiangrial station. It had two safari tents and a grass-roofed tukul. They made a lot of clay bricks and built a classroom for the training center (BELC). Twenty-five students did three years of study there.

## VISIT ONE TO THIANGRIAL IN FEBRUARY 2007

We held a community meeting about safe water to drink. I asked someone to bring me a water sample from the Nile River to look at under a microscope. There were germs in it moving around!

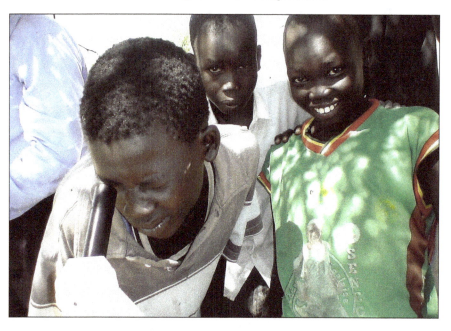

## VISIT TWO TO THIANGRIAL IN OCTOBER 2007

We came with the water purifier system and set it up on the shore of the river.

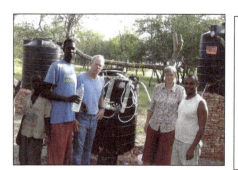

The **Thiangrial community is enjoying clean water** from a new water treatment system. Using a solar-powered submersible pump, river water is pumped into a tank for sedimentation overnight. In a second tank, all germs in the water are killed when simple solar-powered equipment converts common salt to chlorine gas. The water is then pumped into a third tank and is ready to drink. This clean water is available to all the students at our Education Centers as well as Sudanese residents in the surrounding villages. Community participation is important for all of our projects. The Thiangrial community assisted in setting up the system and now keeps it maintained. **This safe drinking water system will now be set up at other bases.**

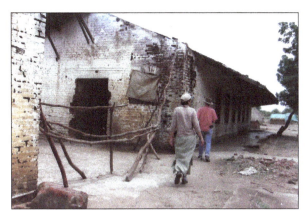

At our first trip to Doro in 2006, we found two old hospital buildings standing, but in very poor condition.

In 2008, major renovations started on the old hospital buildings, thanks to several building teams who came to help out.

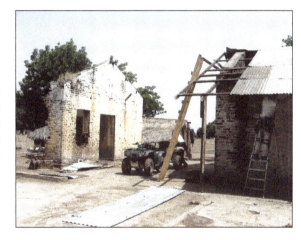

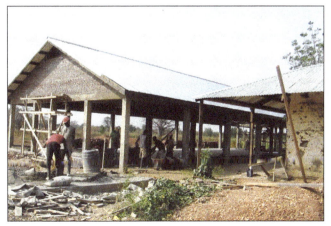

In 2009 work began on a new Maternity Center building beside the old buildings. It would have the capacity to do a C section to save mother and baby.

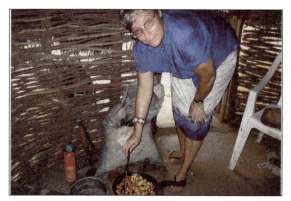

This picture is taken inside Vicki's and my kitchen tukul at Doro. We cooked on charcoal stoves every evening. We could buy charcoal in the local market. AIM AIR pilots did not want to fly in propane gas bottles on flights with passengers.

Learning to cook and bake with a solar cooker was kind of fun.

It was made in Kenya, and I took it to Doro in 2007. The mid-day sun reflected off the raised top. Your dish or cake pan sits under the flat glass cover.

Rice would cook for supper in there if boiling water was used initially to mix with the rice.

The charcoal oven I found in a Kenya market replaced this solar cooker around 2008.

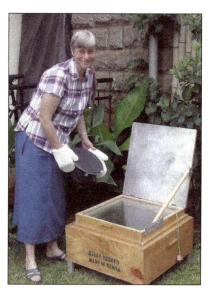

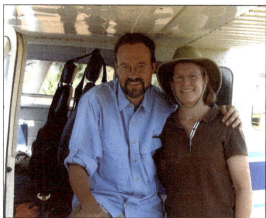

This is Dr. Rob and Nancy Congdon, our team leaders at Doro while I was there.

They are from Oregon. What an incredible job they did to get the health project going and oversee building the whole station! Let alone all the bush doctor work Dr. Rob did at Doro.

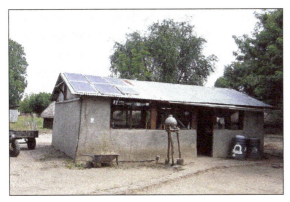

This is our "dining hall" at Doro, which was the center of life on the compound. See the solar panels on the roof, the hand-washing station by the door up on three sticks, and our black water barrels to the right of the door. There is a satellite dish off to the left for our email.

This man and his donkey were paid to deliver water from the community well to our compound barrels.

He filled our barrels up about three times a week.

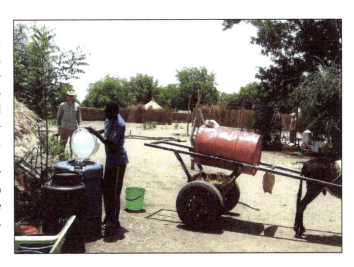

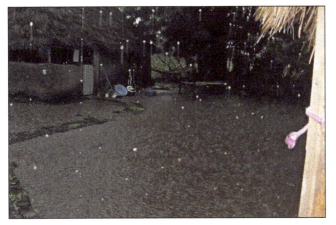

It is pouring rain. See why we had brick sidewalks all over the compound? Rainy season goes from May to November.

## CHAPTER 16

# APRIL 2008 EVENTS AT DORO AND THE PLANE CRASH. CLOSE CALL #4

*On April 1,* 2008, we were shocked when Dr. David Masters died at 5:30 a.m. in his tent at Doro. He had had some diarrhea periodically the previous week, and on the afternoon of March 31, he really felt unwell and weak. Vicki and I had a quick meeting with him about 4:00 p.m. on the thirty-first, and afterwards he said he was going to go lie down. He had no fever, but increasing nausea and abdominal pain from what I heard. I did not get involved that evening because his wife, Irene, was a nurse, and Sandy and Sarah, a physician assistant, were helping.

At 1:00 a.m. I woke and saw lights still on at the Masters's tent. Sandy and Sarah were both there, so I knew he was very sick. When I awoke again at 4:30 a.m. and saw their tent light still on, I decided to get up and see if there was anything I could do to help. Sandy and Irene were there. Sandy said I should retake his blood pressure. I went in and found it to be barely audible at 92 systolic, no diastolic heard. In fact, I could not feel a peripheral pulse, or hear his heart due to his wet breathing. He was gurgling. Sandy kept telling him to slow down his breathing, but his rapid breathing was involuntary.

I suggested to Sandy that she go home and get some rest and she did. Irene and I got David to turn on his side finally. Earlier he would not turn because it hurt his abdomen too much. His abdomen was very distended. David said, "Just let me rest." I thought he might close his eyes and sleep, but a few minutes after we turned him, his eyes rolled back and he was unresponsive.

Oh my! I was scared and I ran to wake up Dr. Angelina, our Sudanese doctor on the base. She came straight away. He was hardly breathing. We pressed his sternum to stimulate breathing. I called out for a manual breathing mask/ bag, nasal-gastric tube, adrenaline, etc., but they could not find anything that we needed. Sarah came in, but he was already gone.

Irene had left him when I ran for Dr. Angelina, and she never came back into the tent. Apparently, at about 4 a.m., just before I arrived, David had told Irene he would not be there in the morning to tell her he loved her. It was the most helpless feeling to watch him die. We never will know for sure what he died of. There was no fever. Later, Dr. Rob said his best guess was that he died of acute bowel obstruction.

As soon as he died, I asked Sandy to get Dr. Rob on the satellite phone. He was on vacation on the coast of Kenya. I told him David had just died. He knew David was very sick because Sandy had phoned him around 1 a.m. for advice, but no one thought he would die. I asked Sandy to get the Sudan director, JoAnn Brant, on the phone and she, or someone, did. JoAnn was at Loki about to board a plane for Renk to attend the Sudan Interior Church executive meeting. Apparently, Dr. Rob had already called her, and she told me that Jimmy Cox would handle things in Nairobi. She also said that David had signed a document saying that if he died in Africa he wanted to be buried in Africa. So she simply said we were to bury him at Doro.

I said, "Well, we can't!" "Why not? What do you mean?" she said.

I kept quiet because I just thought a plane would come. I could not imagine having to bury him right there, that day. Irene remembered David signing something about this, but said she still needed to ask her children before deciding anything. Due to the time change in England, Irene said she would phone her son about 8 a.m. our time. I went back into the tent.

David was a very tall and big man. He was lying way off the foot of the mattress. I asked someone to come in and help me. John, our short-term builder, came and we managed to shift him up to the top of the mattress. His eyes would not stay closed. I removed his IV and started gathering things into one place. Everything was wet, dirty, and strewn all over. It was daybreak. Many were crying. We were all absolutely stunned. Eventually we all went up to the dining hall. Sebsibe said he and Abebe (our Ethiopia missionaries) would ride their bikes to town to report it to the commissioner. I talked to Bob and John Maruti, our builders, about making a coffin. We had only just got some lumber about ten days before this. I said that whether he leaves here on a plane, or is buried here, we would need a coffin today. I phoned

Jimmy and told him Irene had yet to tell her children and decide about burial arrangements. We waited until Irene finally phoned her son. The family concluded that they would respect his wish to be buried right here. Some church leaders had already left for the Renk meetings. We thought our station manager, Nehemiah, had gone too, but he was still home, heard the news in town and came. What a relief to have him there. Jimmy asked Sebsibe, our Ethiopian missionary, to plan the funeral. The team from Yabus SIM station said they were coming over to Doro, which was really nice.

Around 9 a.m. I knew what had to be done. I discreetly asked Sarah to come with me back to David. I told her there was a smell in the tent. We managed to remove all the soiled linens and started to get David dressed in trousers and shirt. When we turned him to his side to get the shirt on, he let go of a lot of clear liquid and groaned (I don't know why). I removed all medical things from the tent. Then I told Irene he was dressed and cleaned up. We asked one young gal to come and wash all the linens. Later on, I kicked myself for not wearing gloves for that job because we didn't know what he died of.

I thought Irene would come and visit him, but she did not want to see him dead. I sat in a chair in the shade outside David's tent for the next three hours or so. Many Mabaan friends and church members began coming to see him and grieve. They were not afraid to touch his body. Our students came. We were all so shocked. Everyone was around Irene a lot. Not one of the missionaries that I am aware of came into the tent to see David.

Vicki sat with me part of the time. At noon Bob and John Maruti came to me and said the tent was too hot for the body. The funeral was set for 4 p.m. I went and got my cot and set it up on the veranda of my new unfinished *tukul* house. The guys moved David on his mattress to my veranda. When I went for lunch, Sandy came and sat with David. Dr. Rob had sent a text message earlier and said he was coming. We did not know when, but it felt right and so good to know he was coming. In fact, he and his wife Nancy came on Friday. David had died early on Tuesday morning.

David Masters is buried in our little cemetery at Doro along with Dr. Bob Grieves and his wife, and a nurse. Our students offered to dig the grave. Someone told me that in the place where they started to dig his grave, they found what looked like a baby's grave, so there were others buried there too with unmarked graves. On the cross grave marker, Nate Kidder from Yabus painted "I have fought a good fight, I have finished the race, I have kept the faith." All I remember at David's burial service was Pastor David saying, "We will not meet David walking on the road again."

I was with David for less than an hour before he died. Many supplies we needed to help him were either not at Doro or maybe up at the new clinic. Dr. Rob later said that even if David had been in a hospital, he probably would not have lived. We all had regrets and thought of what we should have done differently, but we had to let go and accept that God's will was done. It was not anyone's fault that he died.

Dr. David was our station manager at the time. With him gone, by default, I handled many decisions that day and the following three weeks before I was scheduled to leave Doro for seven months of furlough.

This was the third missionary death I had been directly involved with. The first one was in 1977 when our Bembereke Hospital lab tech died of Lassa Fever. The second was in 1994 in Addis Ababa when Andrea Buheital died in pregnancy. And now Dr. David Masters in 2008. All three were very different circumstances, and all three were very tough.

*SATURDAY, APRIL 26, 2008 AT DORO*

We were not even supposed to be flying that day. Sandy and I had booked a plane to leave on the next Tuesday. But on Friday afternoon, Sandy received a satellite phone message from Nairobi that we were to prepare to leave the next morning, which was Saturday, April 26. I was most unhappy about that because it meant quick packing up for furlough, saying goodbyes, and leaving many things undone at school.

The plane arrived about 9 a.m. Saturday morning. Just as the pilot landed at Doro, it started to rain. Debbie Sardo and Claire Meckler were passengers on the flight and came over to our dining hall on the station to wait for the rain to stop. The pilot stayed out on the airstrip with the plane. The airstrip at Doro was dirt. By the time the pilot unloaded our cargo and fueled up the plane, it was still raining and they do not take off in rain. We enjoyed a good visit for about three hours while it rained that morning. We thought it would prevent us from leaving that day. I remember saying to the pilot, "Let's not take any chances," but about noon he wanted to take off. It was VERY muddy. I sank down in mud so deep that my tennis shoes were covered in mud just from walking out to the airstrip. I had to remove my shoes at the top of the ladder in the plane. I sat down with just socks on. I said to Sandy about three times as we taxied to the end of the airstrip, "We shouldn't be doing this. It is too muddy." And she said to me, "It's the pilot's call. He knows."

The pilot told us we would not be able to make it all the way to Nairobi now, but that the plane had to get to Loki, Kenya, tonight. The pilot was in a hurry. And there was no way I was going to be left behind. I was truly tired of everything at Doro and wanted to leave for furlough. The bottom line is that I got on that plane of my own free will.

When we started down the muddy airstrip, alarm sounds were going off in the plane before we got airborne. We did get up to about treetop height, but, without enough speed, the plane went into an aerodynamic stall. It came back down to the ground and we were crashing forward through small tree stuff very fast. I remember bracing myself with my left hand on the back of the pilot's seat and thinking we were truly going to crash and die. I was in the middle seat of three seats behind the pilot. Then we were upside down because the plane had gone into a gully and flipped over on its nose! I managed to release my seat belt and fell down onto all fours. I got up on my knees.

The pilot was already out looking at the plane, saying, "Oh it's bad!"

Debbie, on my left, was crying out with pain. Sandy, on my right, said, "I smell gas."

We were afraid of fire! So I told Debbie I was going to release her seat belt because we had to get out of there as fast as we could! Debbie fell down on all fours. "My neck hurts," she cried out. She did not get up.

I turned to my right and tried to release Sandy, but could not. Her seat belt release was under something. I tried twice, but it hurt my chest to reach up and try very hard. I told Sandy I could not undo it. Claire had released herself in the seat behind us. I think I asked Claire to help Debbie get out. Debbie crawled away from the plane in the mud. I said to Sandy, "I'm not leaving you, Sandy. I'm sure Ray will be here any minute to help us." She became unconscious with a beet red face as she hung upside down.

Soon someone came to help. He was a big Sudanese man. I got out in order to give him space to get in and help Sandy. He came back out after a minute or so and said, "I need a knife to cut the seatbelt." I guess the pilot had one on his belt. Soon the man was carrying Sandy out.

I went to sit beside Debbie and Claire not far from the plane. It was raining again. We all sat or lay in the mud. It soon became clear that Claire was not all right. She had been hovering over Debbie and kept asking us the same questions of where were we, what happened, who was there, etc. I finally told Claire to lie down because she was disoriented and could not remember anything that had just happened. Later I saw the bruise on her right temple area. She complained of numbness and tingling down her arms. Those were alarming symptoms.

I had cried for a bit after the crash—it was all so frightening. The back of my left hand was swollen. My chest hurt and I could not lie down. I just sat there and talked to Debbie and Claire. I asked Debbie if it hurt more in the front or back of her neck. And she said in front and down the right shoulder, which relieved me a bit.

Amy arrived from the station and came to us, crying. I looked Amy in the eye and said we should get some cervical collars for both of them before moving them. Amy came around and stopped crying. Ray came and asked me if I was all right. I told him my chest hurt. All of us had chest pains. A number of people were around Sandy, who was a bit away from us. I thought she must be hurt badly, and, indeed, her unconsciousness was a huge concern.

One by one, they began taking us back to the station in the trailer behind the 4-wheeler. I remember a tractor came from somewhere but could not get up the muddy slope. It tried and tried. I started to shiver because I was soaking wet and sitting on the muddy ground. It seemed about an hour before they said it was my turn to leave. Bob was there with the 4-wheeler and trailer to take me back to the station. I got up on my knees, and with help, I managed to stand up. I had no shoes on. I sat in the trailer and tried to lie back but could not breathe, it hurt so. Abebech, one of our Ethiopian missionaries, got in and I leaned back on her for support for the ride back to the station.

Wodenesh, another of the Ethiopian missionaries, sat at my feet. Bob almost did not get up one muddy slope. I had no idea where we were.

When we finally arrived at the station, they put me in Vicki's *tukul*. Abebech and Wodenesh took off my wet clothes and dressed me in their own dry clothes because all of my things were packed away. They placed a warm blanket around me, and then Wodenesh came with some warm water in a pan and put my feet in it. Oh, that felt good.

I was being left alone off and on because Vicki and Wodenesh and Abebech were in and out of the *tukul* getting things or talking on the satellite phone. At one point I told Vicki to please not leave me alone. I was still scared. Soon Lloyd came in to sit with me. He told me what he thought happened out there. Being from Alaska, he knew planes. He said we hit a gully and the plane had flipped.

After some time, I told Vicki and Lloyd I felt woozy and started to get hot. Either I did pass out or almost did. My blood pressure had dropped. They told Dr. Rob by phone and he said I must lie down and to start an IV. I objected to lying down, but somehow they got me from the chair to the bed. I could not lie down. I was crying with chest pain, which was caused by muscle spasms in my left side. Abebech got behind me again on the bed and I leaned on her. At some point Anne Lee came in and told me that Esther (the Kenyan United Nations director in charge of repatriation of refugees) was calling in a UN helicopter to medically evacuate us all to a UN hospital in Malakal (on the Nile River). What a relief to be able to get out where there was more help for all of us.

It was about 6 p.m. when the helicopter arrived. I was in misery with an IV that was not working in my right wrist, and pain in my left hand. Amy had checked my ribs and listened to my chest, but she could not find the problem. It started to become clear to me later on that it was my sternum that was injured, not my ribs. Any movement caused spasms. Somehow they got me back in a chair and lifted the whole chair to the trailer outside the door. Then they lifted me from the trailer to the back of a Land Cruiser, and I sat on a stretcher.

The cruiser got stuck in a big mud hole on its way to the airstrip. The driver was rocking the vehicle to get out until I told him to please stop. The jerking was hurting too much. So another vehicle backed up to us and they moved my stretcher over to it. Finally, we got to the end of the airstrip where the helicopter was. It was almost dark.

One U.N. guy came over to me and he pressed on my sternum! Oh my goodness I nearly passed out, and if I could have, I think I would have kicked the guy. I remember asking one of the medical people there to take out the IV because it was not working. Dr. Angelina said she did not want to remove it without gloves. I remember telling her that I did not have HIV. Someone did remove the IV. They finally lifted my chair onto the helicopter. Inside someone listened to my chest. And then I managed to get over to a comfortable seat. I deliberately closed my eyes for about an hour. I did not want to talk to anyone. I did not want to see us going up in the air. I had earphones on because it was very noisy. I wanted to be left alone. I prayed. I did not sleep, but just got myself relaxed, and by not moving an inch, the pain went away. After about an hour I opened my eyes and looked around. It was very dark outside the window and raining.

The India contingent of the United Nations runs a makeshift hospital in Malakal, on the Nile River. We arrived in the ward about 10 p.m. Andrew (our SIMer living in Malakal) was there to meet us. The pilot, Claire, and I were in one ward, which was set up in a forty-foot shipping container. We did not see Debbie and Sandy until morning. The Indian doctor had a head turban on. He did not exam me. He asked me a few questions. All three of us got an IV started, a tetanus shot, and a pain shot. I wonder if the doctor did not do a physical exam because we were women and Christian besides. Later, Sandy and I compared notes, and they had the same general treatments and no physical exam. Around midnight they kindly brought in some Indian food, but I could not eat. My biggest problem that night was that the head of my stretcher would not go up. It was a long night of mostly sitting up with nothing to lean on. Around the middle of the night I happened to notice a huge seatbelt bruise across my lower abdomen from hip to hip with an abrasion on one end. I really wondered what all was wrong with me. The pain shot had helped considerably, but eventually it wore off. Nevertheless, I was very grateful to be out of Doro.

They did an X-ray of my chest and hand at Malakal. The AP (frontal) view of the chest X-ray showed no fractures. They said my hand had a dislocation, not a fracture. That was correct. Only the chest lateral (side) view in Nairobi showed the sternum fracture, so we did not know it was broken until I got to the hospital in Nairobi.

Around noon on Sunday the AIM AIR plane arrived in Malakal to get us. It was the big DC 3 plane. I was never so glad to see Dr. Rob Congdon as that day. He checked us all out. After listening to my lungs, he said that he was very happy. No lung puncture.

It was very significant and a great blessing to be med-evacuated out of Doro that day. After watching Dr. David die at Doro on a dark night in a hot tent with no pain medicine or the help he needed, I know that's why I was afraid for myself and the others. Vicki, Ray and Ann, Amy, and Angelina did not want us spending the night in Doro, either. I don't know when the airstrip would have been dried out enough for an airplane to have landed at Doro to get us. Only a helicopter could evacuate us that day. It was good that Sandy and I had been attending all the U.N. meetings in town and had good connections with Esther, the coordinator of the U.N. repatriation program. Esther had the clout to call in the U.N. helicopter for us. I will forever be grateful for the U.N. humanitarian help.

God did help us through a very tough day and week. I stayed at the Congdons' house for a week after spending one night at Nairobi Hospital. On April 30, Dr. Louis Carter operated on my hand. Dr. Carter is a retired SIM doctor who was visiting Kijabe hospital for six weeks. Incredibly, he was there and was able to pin the dislocated metacarpal joint in my hand. He was very kind. The AIM orthopedic doctor, Dr. Tim Mead, had a sister in Grand Rapids, Michigan, who agreed to see me for follow-up on my hand. There were two pins in that joint and they needed to be removed in five weeks. In all, I was in Nairobi for three weeks before I flew home for furlough. Dr. Rob went to Doro about a week after the plane crash for a few days. He brought back letters. Each of the students had written me a precious note, which I have kept. Somehow Ruth Clark was able to get the Congdons' phone number where I was staying to recover, and Ruth called me, which was really nice. The plane crash investigators took me out to lunch one day in Nairobi and asked me to describe in detail what I remembered. That was really the last I heard from AIM AIR.

How did my family find out about the plane crash? Well, that is worth telling. Hours after the plane crash on that Saturday, our Sudan director, JoAnn Brant, sent out an email to many SIM people, including Jim Mason in Canada. Jim was a friend of Pastor Peter DeKlerk at Calvary Bible Church in Lapeer, Michigan. Pastor Peter announced to their Sunday evening service audience that I had been in a plane crash and to pray. Their evening service was broadcast over a Christian radio station (WMPC). One listener heard that I was injured and called my cousin to ask how Barb was. My cousin did not know anything about it. He called my brother Robert. Robert didn't know anything about it either. Robert called JoAnn Brandt in Nairobi and learned what happened. When JoAnn came to the hospital early Monday to see me, she immediately handed me her phone and said to call my brother right away, explaining that he had called her and was pretty upset to not have been informed by the mission of the plane crash. I talked to Robert that day and about every day that week, except the day of my hand surgery. My family was thinking, "Here we go again."

It is no small thing that God mercifully saved our lives. It did not take me long to compare this terrible day to the night Dr. David died. There were no miracles that night. It is clearly not always God's will to deliver us from danger and death. Ours is to pray, "Lord, I will trust you—no matter what." For God is trustworthy no matter what kind of crises we are going through. Jesus said, "In this world you will face trouble, but be encouraged, I have overcome the world." That is why I have titled these memoirs as an assignment to trust God, whether He delivers us from danger and death, or not. Some people turn away from God when the going gets tough, others turn to God, and rise above hard things. Let us go with God.

## Summary of the Plane Crash Miracles

1.  Upon the aerodynamic stall of the plane at treetop height, it came down to earth, and we were soon off the end of the muddy airstrip. We crashed through the bush, miraculously just missing a baobab tree in our path to the gully. The very tip of the right wing actually did break off somewhere in the bush. The wings were full of fuel.
2.  That the plane flipped from nose to tail and not sideways is a miracle. The wings were full of fuel and would have exploded if we had flipped sideways.
3.  A large Sudanese man was the first person to arrive to help. I backed out of the plane. He soon came back out and asked for a knife. The pilot had one and gave it to him. He cut Sandy's seat

belt to free her and carried her out of the plane. He returned the knife to the pilot and we never saw him again. We do not know his name. He spoke good English too. I believe he was a guardian angel sent by God to help! I really do!

4. The four-wheel ATV and trailer had been at Doro only two weeks. We were evacuated one at a time from the plane crash site back to the station in the trailer behind the ATV. No other vehicle would have been able to get through the mud.

5. Esther, in charge of UN repatriation, was in Bunj (three miles from Doro) that weekend. She came to Doro, and seeing Sandy and me, who had attended all of the U.N. meetings for SIM, she called on her satellite phone to U.N. headquarters and requested a helicopter be sent to Doro as soon as possible to evacuate all five injured passengers. No one else could have gotten us out of Doro that day!

6. No one was sure what was wrong with my left hand. I could not move my thumb and my hand was swollen below the thumb. By God's grace, Dr. Louis Carter was at Kijabe Hospital for a six-week stint. He was a skilled hand surgeon and retired SIM Nigeria doctor. I knew him by reputation. He and his wife had two weeks to go in their planned six-week visit in Kenya. He did not really need the X-ray. He just examined my hand and immediately diagnosed a left first metacarpal dorsal dislocation of the joint. He operated on my hand two days later. Two pins were placed using a fluoroscopic type of machine to see the joint, as opposed to an incision, and the pins held the joint in place for five weeks of healing. My ticket home, booked in January, went to Detroit on May 16–17. I was able to use that ticket home and made it to my niece Rachel's high school graduation!

# Just a Short-Term Trip?
### by Rob Congdon, from the U.S., working in Sudan

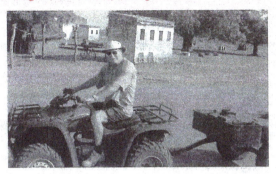

Last May I returned to Doro to help at the increasingly busy medical clinic, to meet with community and church leaders to plan for the future, and to advise four wonderful builders from Canada and Alaska who came to lend a hand during this critical period of time. They put the finishing touches on a concrete-block storage shed just in time for the rainy season. Repairs were made to pit latrines and showers, and they finished three additional thatch huts for living quarters. The lone usable building at the old hospital site is cleaned and occupied,

But the team returned home with more memories than simply the 120° F. heat and complicated engineering challenges. They won't forget how through tears they hammered together a rough wooden casket for David Masters; how they ran with hearts pounding down the airstrip toward a mangled, flipped-over plane; how they welcomed thousands of returning refugees brought by open truck from Ethiopian camps; and how they shared the Good News joyfully in classroom devotional times and church gatherings. ◾

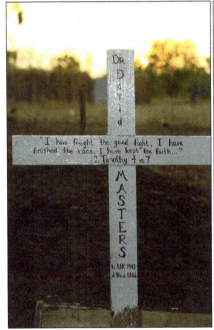

"I have fought the good fight, I have finished the race, I have kept the faith..."
2 Timothy 4 vs 7

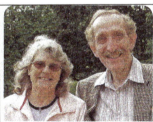

# Sudan team loses much-loved "bush doctor"

>> "If I 'sleep' in Sudan, bury me in Sudan," requested David Masters, a bush doctor serving with the Rebuilding Southern Sudan team. After a medical career in Congo and the U.K., he and his wife Irene "retired" to serve at Doro, Sudan. After only two months there, following an active day of treating patients, he developed severe abdominal pain and a high fever and died within hours. Meanwhile, over the past couple of years, the Sudan team has grown to about 60 people, and together they are seeing people respond to the Gospel and gather to worship Jesus. They're also providing safe water and health care.

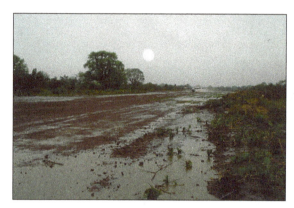

April 26, 2008.

12:30 p.m.

That is our Cessna 208 (caravan) plane coming down Doro airstrip for takeoff. It's too muddy. It went up to treetop height, but went into an aerodynamic stall and came down.

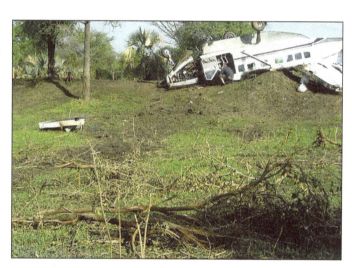

We flipped over in a gully, landing upside down with tires up in the air.

If it had rolled sideways, it probably would have caught fire, as the fuel is in the wings.

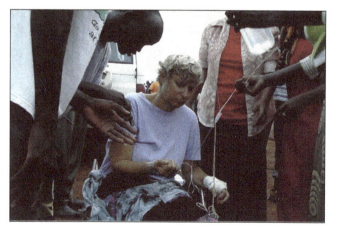

I was miserable and in pain with a fractured sternum.

This picture was taken as I was carried in a chair onto the UN helicopter for evacuation to Malakal on the Nile River.

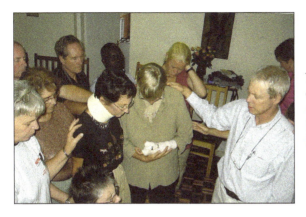

Ten days after the plane crash, our Sudan team met for a prayer meeting in Nairobi, Kenya, at our headquarters.

Us four ladies pictured here three weeks after the plane crash, in fact, the day I left Nairobi to go home:

Debbie Sardo
Sandy Ewan
Claire Meckler and
myself

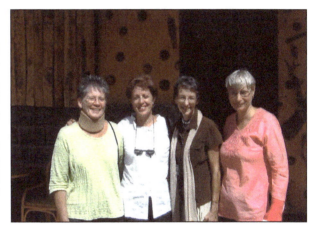

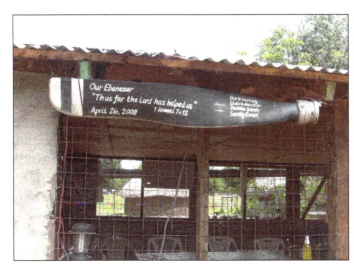

The souvenir propeller blade hung on our dining room rafters as "Our Ebenezer" to remember God's help that day.

193

CHAPTER 17

# THE COMMUNITY HEALTH WORKER
# SCHOOL AT DORO (2008–2010)

*Determined to return* to Doro as planned in January 2009, I stoically boarded an AIM AIR airplane in Nairobi, Kenya, and flew to Doro for my second term in South Sudan. All four passengers who had been in the plane crash went back to South Sudan. We would not be deterred by the enemy and God's work went forward.

Vicki had conducted the application and interview process and selected a new class of twelve students for our 2009 class of community health workers. I left my mother living with my sister and put home and Hadley behind me. Plans were to teach the nine-month, government-approved CHW Course in 2009 and again in 2010. I told my family I would be back in 2011 and then pray about my future plans. We had a rule as a family, which was, if you start a game—you finish it. I would not let the plane crash and whatever fears my family or I had keep me from finishing my five-year commitment to God and to the South Sudan team. I worked hard to get the school going and I liked the work very much.

A couple of weeks after I returned to Doro, Dave Bremner visited us. He was our SIM International Deputy Director in charge of East Africa ministries. He asked me if I had revisited the site of the plane crash. I said, "No, I have not." He said, "We need to do that." So he and Chris Crowder (our Sudan director), Vicki, Sarah Benson, Sandy Ewan, and I walked down to the airstrip and off the end of it to the gully where the plane had flipped over. AIM AIR had picked up every bit of the broken plane and taken it back to Nairobi. On the way there, they pointed out to me the baobab tree we had just missed. They pointed out another tree, which they believe the tip of one wing hit, so fuel ran out of the end of that wing instead of toward the engine, avoiding a deadly fire. Chris read from Psalm 121 and Dave prayed as we held hands in a circle on site. Indeed, we remembered many miracles and we thanked God for them. It was a good experience and sort of a closure to that event.

The propeller blade that had broken off was retrieved, and Sandy requested it from AIM AIR. We hung the blade from the rafters of our dining room at Doro for all to remember God's mercy. Painted on it were these words: Our Ebenezer, "Thus far the Lord has helped us," I Samuel 7:12; April 26, 2008; Barb Hartwig, Claire Meckler, Debbie Sardo, Sandy Ewan."

I would add that Dave Bremner had been our speaker at our first Sudan Spiritual Life Conference for the new Sudan team two years earlier. It was held in Loki (Kenya) in January 2007, and he gave daily Bible teaching from the book of Daniel. I have good notes from his teaching and will quote what Dave had said about Daniel, chapter three (the fiery furnace): "King Nebuchadnezzar was angry. What God can rescue you from my hand? God is able, but even if not . . . Faith that is proved genuine is glory to God. God leads us into difficulties while we try to avoid them. See the miracle that follows a predicament. When God brings adversity, it is for us to persevere. Will God find faith in you? Your faith is of great value to God." That lesson applied to all of us involved with Dr. David's death and the plane crash in April of 2008. But remember this—there were no miracles or special helps the night Dr. David died in his hot tent. Thus genuine faith cannot be dependent on miracles and happy outcomes.

While I did not like flying in small planes in and out of South Sudan after the plane crash, I would like to record one particular flight on 9/25/2009 out of Doro to Kenya. The pilot that day was AIM AIR's Jim Streit (head pilot at that time). When he landed at Doro, Jim explained that when he saw Sandy Ewan, Debbie Sardo, and me, all on the passenger list, he requested the flight. He surprised us with seats at the front of the plane and he had removed the copilot seat in order to interact with us better in-flight. He gave us headsets so that the four of us could communicate easily. When he kindly handed me some cheese crackers and oranges to share among us, I shed tears. Unless you have lived without such food for months, you probably cannot appreciate how special that tasted. He took the plane up high, and God provided beautiful white and gray clouds with a bright blue sky background that day. It was the most beautiful sight I have ever seen on a flight. Another God-moment "up there" was when Jim played Kathy Troccoli's song *Go Light Your World,* one of my favorite songs. I definitely experienced healing in my mind and spirit that special day way up there in the clouds.

As if that was not special enough, Jim and his wife also took us out to dinner in Nairobi! It was the first and only time AIM AIR really recognized us, and yet, no one even mentioned the plane crash during the flight or at dinner. What that was all about, I don't know for sure, but isn't it good to remember and recognize those who were hurt, recovered, returned, and did not blame.

Back to business, we were about one month into the training course when on Thursday evening, March 5, 2009, I hurried to the dining hall to quickly send my nephew Chad a happy birthday email. When I opened up my email I saw an urgent message from my sister-in-law Tamra telling me that mom had had a severe heart attack at my sister's house on March 3. They had brought her back home by ambulance to our local hospital and she was not expected to live. My heart sank after reading that email. I talked it over with my colleagues that night and decided to go home for three weeks.

The soonest I could get a flight back to Kenya was on Saturday. I flew out of Nairobi on Sunday evening and reached mom's bedside on Monday evening. She knew me and, in fact, rallied a bit. I spent every day with her. She was very weak and did not want to get out of bed. Finally, we all agreed to move her to inpatient hospice care, about seven miles from our home.

On March 31 I still did not know what to do. My return ticket was for April 1. I had until noon on March 31 to change the ticket. We got a phone call that morning that my Uncle Bob Hartwig had just died. My mother did not want me to go. Ruth Clark did not think I should go yet, either. So I rebooked my ticket and stayed another three weeks. It is a good thing I did. The evening of March 31, I received an email from Vicki saying they had had to close the school at Doro because five Dinka students needed personal leave to go home for something. They were given twenty days leave and told school would reopen on April 20. My ticket to Nairobi was on April 22. Wow! God's time is the best time and He did lead me that last day of March, so I got to spend three more weeks with Mom.

April 21 was my last day with Mom. I spent seven hours at her bed-side. We didn't really talk much. Leaving, I told her I loved her and we both had tears. We both knew I had to go and we knew that I would miss her funeral. She supported me throughout my missionary days and will receive whatever jewels in heaven there are for her staunch support and help. My ten-year-old niece wrote this in a book in the chapel at the Goodrich Hospice: "May everyone here be blessed as a Christian. I hope they all had a good life. I know Grandma H. did. I am blessed to have her. Thank you, God, Briana Hartwig." Ditto, Briana! Mom died on May 14, 2009, about three weeks after I left her.

Classes resumed at the school, and we still managed to finish the class of 2009 in November by not taking any more breaks that year. The year of 2009 proved to be a time of building up at Doro. A new maternity center building was begun that would enable doctors to do a cesarean section operation to save lives. This big building project required a lot of supplies, logistics, and both hired workers and vis-iting building teams. I was treasurer at Doro that year, which meant I had to keep cash on hand to pay wages, and building supplies for the station. Keeping the school account and station account and personal money straight was a big job, especially when I had to do it in three different currencies. Kenya shillings, Sudanese pounds, and American dollars were used by everyone.

Why were we specifically building a maternity center? Here is a statistic about South Sudan that is staggering. The maternal, meaning pregnant women, mortality rate was 2,037 deaths per 100,000 women. It was said to be the highest in the world. Compare that to 800 deaths per 100,000 women in Kenya and 12 deaths per 100,000 women in the USA. And another sad statistic was that one out of five under-five year-old kids would die. There was a lot of work to do in health care for the families of southern Sudan. That is why the training of tradi-tional birth attendants, which Vicki and I called our trained had done the year before, was so important. It was these grandmothers who did home deliveries and were trained to recognize complications and refer the pregnant woman to the hospital when necessary. Vicki and I called our trained TBAs together for a meeting three times a year for supervision and encouragement.

We had some fun at school one afternoon. It was during our lesson about doing a physical exam. I asked the students to invite all the under-five-year-old kids they could find to come to our classroom at 3 p.m. that afternoon. Now after consistently shooing away little curious kids around our classroom, this was a switch. This would be our practical exercise doing head-to-toe exams. Around twenty-five kids came very happily to class. We had mats on the floor for them to sit down. Mothers were standing by or else did not come. We gave each child a piece of candy to begin with, and the students explained in the Mabaan language what we were doing. I paired up the students and gave each pair something to assess. For example, two students assessed the skin condition of each child. Another pair of students assessed each child's eyes for anemia and anything abnormal. Another pair of students checked their abdomen for any signs of sickness. When all was said and done, we sent the kids home and compared notes. A couple of the kids had multiple problems, and I asked the Mabaan students to follow up with a home visit to talk with the mothers.

My home church collected money for mosquito nets, thanks to an initiative by Robin McIlroy. If I remember right, around $700 was collected, and I spent that money in Nairobi, where I found a good deal on hundreds of mosquito nets. The students, along with Vicki and me, went to two villages by tractor and wagon for practical experience in community health work. We went to Gasmalla village one day each in April, May and June, having sent a letter ahead notifying them of our coming. Upon arriving in the villages, our group would greet the chief and then find two big trees to work under. Mothers, babies, and kids arrived to hear a devotional talk and prayer to begin the day. We weighed every baby and child and recorded it on their "Road To Health" card. We taught the students how to graph the weight for age and see if the "dot" fell within the normal weight for age. We were looking for malnourished kids. The student would talk with the mother about what she was feeding her child, be it breastfeeding or weaning foods or regular foods. Each mother who came would receive a mosquito net. We demonstrated how to set it up and explained the value of using it. This was to prevent malaria from nocturnal mosquito bites. There was a lot of talking and weighing and advice going around while we were there.

My days were full. I was up at 6 a.m. with my personal devotions and breakfast finished before 7 a.m., Monday through Friday, with a 10–15 minute prayer meeting together in the dining room. Everyone was expected to be there. We took turns leading it. It was also a good time for any station announcement that needed to be made. By 2009 there were around fifteen missionaries living at Doro. Dr. Rob Congdon was in charge. He and Nancy and their six sons lived in Kenya, but Rob made frequent trips to Doro and would stay one to two weeks at a time. The leadership team at Doro included Dr. Rob, Sandy Ewan (in charge of the clinic), Vicki Beattie (in charge of community outreach), and myself (in charge of the CHW training school). By 7:30 I was at our school office and made a shopping list for our daily town-tripper guy (employee) to go by bike to the market and buy food and supplies. At 8 a.m. class started, and I led devotions and prayers with the students for thirty minutes. We did a chronological walk through the Bible with the Gospel Recording picture books. Let me mention that at our 2010 graduation I was able to purchase a set of these nine picture books for each graduate with gift money from my home church's Rex Curtiss missions fund. The late Rex Curtiss would have liked that. Class ran from 8:30 a.m. to noon each day and sometimes in the afternoon. I gave homework, prepared quizzes and tests, and expected a lot from the students. They were eager to learn and most of them did well, considering their varied educational backgrounds. After lunch break at our compound, I routinely went back to the office and prepared for the next days' lessons. In 2009 Vicki did less and less classroom teaching and more community outreach. In 2010 Vicki was doing the leprosy treatment program full time, and I handled the school load by myself.

Let me put into succinct phrases what daily life at Doro was like:

- Fill the water filter in my *tukul*
- Hand wash all my clothes, sheets and towels on Saturday morning
- In lieu of a bathroom sink, brushing my teeth outside my *tukul*, just leaning over the ground
- Listening to the BBC news every evening
- Filling my thermos in the evening for morning coffee
- One solar panel and inverter at my *tukul* thanks to a Ralph Corey memorial gift
- Email by satellite dish
- Using a mosquito net
- Reading by flashlight at night inside my mosquito net

- Hearing live creature sounds up above the plastic lining of my grass roof
- "Bat pee" is drizzling rain
- Friday night compound movie together if we have enough power in our solar batteries
- Saturday night compound soup and cornbread together
- Sunday night compound devotions together
- Cooking and baking with local charcoal stoves and a charcoal oven
- Three-hour Mabaan church service on Sunday mornings
- Lunch club with daily food in covered dishes in the dining hall from noon to 3 p.m.
- Using my Thuraya satellite phone to call home or Nairobi
- Beware of scorpions, snakes, spiders, army ants, centipedes
- Riding a bike two plus miles to town market for a cold Coke in the open market
- Making brick sidewalks across the compound to walk on due to deep mud in rainy season
- Safari tents and grass *tukuls*
- Pit latrines
- Caleb and Bethany (age 2 and 5) playing with the Sudanese kids
- Keeping the supply up of Plumpy Nut ( a high protein peanut butter-based food at the nutrition center)
- Leprosy drugs from Juba
- Cooking for visiting building teams
- A "send the rubber airplane" kind of day (when you think you are going crazy)
- "Anybody seen Nehemiah?" (our station liaison manager)
- Fiery arrows/shield of faith
- John Maruti requesting the song "You Are My All in All"
- Station meetings to reassign chores; everybody please volunteer for something
- having a feast consisting of goat meat grilled over a pit fire

I liked cooking at Doro. Vicki and I shared a kitchen *tukul*. We each kept a metal trunk with our food and dishes stored in it. About 4:30 or 5 p.m., I would start some charcoal with kerosene. I turned on my little shortwave radio to BBC for world news. It took about thirty minutes for the coals to really get hot. If I was using the charcoal oven, I would put red hot coals on top of black cold coals to get it going. Having homemade desserts did a lot to boost morale, believe it or not. I made a lot of desserts and put them in the dining hall for all to share. My Grandma's fry cakes were very popular on Saturdays. Around 6 p.m. I would take my turn in a bathhouse. That means taking clean clothes, a bucket of water from a barrel, my soap and shampoo and towel. Just a cup and bucket of water was all I used. Back in my *tukul* after a bucket bath, I would sit on my verandah and read with a hand fan going in one hand, a drink in the other, and book on my lap! I was reading through the Bible in two years and enjoyed that quiet, cool relaxed evening read after supper.

Lunch club was a big help to everyone. If you wanted to join this club, you paid cash into a kitty, and we ladies took turns being in charge of organizing the lunch. We hired a Sudanese lady named Tabitha to cook "lunch club" food for us six days a week. The missionary in charge would lay out on the table in the lunch club kitchen *tukul* what Tabitha was to cook that day. By 12:30 she would have it all prepared and hot in covered dishes on the tables in the dining room. Everyone could come and eat anytime between 12:30 and about 3 p.m., when another person would put the leftover food away and wash dishes. At station meetings we all signed up for a chore or two for the good of the station. There were lunch club jobs, cleaning latrine jobs, water jobs, getting daily bread from the market, keeping the hand washing stations filled with water and soap for hand washing, etc. It worked pretty well.

Mary was our cook at the school. Six days a week she cooked three meals for the twelve students, and the students liked her. Mary was shy, she was a Christian, did not know any English, and did not know how to read or write. She had several small children and yet managed to do this job all three years that we ran the school! I paid her weekly, and she would put her thumbprint with ink on a receipt as my record of paying her. One day towards the end of my time there in 2010, I quickly went out to her kitchen tukul to pay her, and when I opened the ink pad for her thumb print, she instead took the pen in my hand and slowly wrote an M on the receipt! I will never forget the look of shy pride on her face when she wrote M! I smiled and complimented her the best that I could in Mabaan words. Someone was teaching her some literacy.

I must relate another student compound story to you. When we started the 2010 school year in February, I knew that the students' *tukuls* needed new grass roofs. We had built them in 2008, and now most would be leaking when the rains came in April. It takes a certain river grass for roofing. One day after class in April, I told the students that I would buy the new grass for the six *tukuls* they lived in, but I asked them to do the work of taking off the old grass and laying the new grass. I said I would pay them sixty sp (Sudanese pounds) per roof for their work, which was the going rate. And I would not have any afternoon classes or give them any homework until the work was done. Some of them were upset and wanted me to hire someone from outside to do the work, but it was urgent that we get started with this. I explained something else to them. We did not charge them tuition or room or board for the whole nine months of the course. Those who came from afar had to pay their own travel, but free tuition and room and board were no small benefit. They all had a wife and kids back home. If they wanted some pocket money, I allowed them to ask for work on either a Friday afternoon or a Saturday from any missionary. I told them that they should see this roofing labor as gratitude work for the education they were receiving. I told them to go and discuss it and give me their answer in the morning. Either it would be leaky roofs this rainy season, or together we would get the job done as soon as possible ourselves.

I wish I could have been a little mouse in the corner listening to their discussion that afternoon. The next morning after devotions I asked them what their decision was. They said I should buy the grass, a short and sweet answer. No further discussion. I arranged through Nehemiah for the grass bundles to be delivered by tractor and wagon. Nehemiah bought the rubber ties in the market and the students went right to work, one *tukul* at a time. At the end, they had enough grass left to also do the kitchen. I paid them one total sum and let them divide it out among themselves. I did not supervise or watch them work, but I could peek at them through the office window. I did notice they seemed happy enough working away, and they finished the whole job a lot sooner than I thought they would. No one can make someone be grateful, but I hope they did it with a heart of gratefulness to God and SIM for the education they were receiving.

On Sunday mornings I attended church right there at Doro. It often was not interpreted to English, so I found it difficult to follow and to worship as I should have. I asked the church leaders if I could start a Sunday school class for the youth. They agreed and gave me an interpreter and wanted it during the sermon time. We did this for about a year. Not one of the young people could read or write. How sad. It made me realize how much I have taken for granted in my life, such as being able to read, and like them, I grew up in the country-side (not a city where more schools are) and was a girl, more unlikely to go to school than boys, but I went to school and learned to read. I had my own Bible, and it was translated into my mother tongue, English. I have had Sunday School teaching and heard sermons and even attended Bible College to help me learn what was in the Bible. It made me grateful for something I had taken for granted all my life.

The class of 2010 turned out to be our best class of the three. By then, the learning curve had done its job, and we knew how to select students; the curriculum was tried and improved; the schedule ran smoothly; and there was no plane crash or mother's death to deal with during the course. We had to expel two students, but eleven graduated. So why stop and go home now?

I will try to explain my reasons in these few words:

- I had finished my five-year commitment to the South Sudan team.
- The government of South Sudan sent out a notice, which I received the day before graduation in November saying that all CHW training was to be suspended until further notice. See a copy of this at the end of this chapter.
- There were uncertainties around the referendum vote coming up and projected independence to be declared by South Sudan in 2011.
- I had no Mabaan language skills, nor was I willing to do formal language learning, which any long-term worker should do.
- I felt wear and tear on body, mind, and soul after five years of this assignment.
- I admitted to being homesick for my family and had certain family responsibilities back home.
- I did not like flying in airplanes anymore, though I did it anyway.

- I was a bit weary of cross-cultural ministry, but not weary of Christian ministry itself.
- Most importantly, because I had prayed and prayed and felt it was God's will at this time to leave.

It was so nice that Tohru and Claire Inoue were at Doro for the graduation in 2010 and for my farewell at Doro. I wanted to have a bonfire and dinner and just sing-a-long with Tohru and his guitar on my last evening. The next day I got on an AIM AIR plane at Doro for the last time and said good-byes to friends and fellow missionaries.

*My first SIM South Sudan field director was Laui, who wrote this poem about life in Sudan. Laui and his wife, Debbie, are from India and put into words very succinctly why we go to this hinterland.*

# For His Love

*by Laui Fachhai, SIM's newest missionary to Sudan*

We do not come here out of mere zest
Life here is not easy at best
Dust, dust, everywhere
Suspicious eyes here and there
Scorching heat, desert storm, malaria
False accusation, opposition, filaria
The cup we're drinking is a bit bitter
 we feel
When we think of others enjoying
 their sweet music reel

Howbeit, we're here because we love
 the Lord
Not because invited but sent by the
 Lord
We choose this for His love leaves us
 no other choice
We come here for we hear and obey
 His voice
A reminder from the Holy Spirit
A renewal of the right spirit
To help us joy in our suffering
To give us strength in difficulties arising

And we thank our Lord for His sufficient grace
Our daily strength and comfort in this
 place

---

### WHEN A TENT IS YOUR HOME...

*... there's no room for a sofa & television.. Well then, what are the essential items for missionary life in southern Sudan? A few of the must-haves are: a large water storage drum, water filter, mosquito net for the bed, durable flashlight, charcoal-burner for cooking, a few pots & dishes, a large washtub for doing laundry and a satellite phone for communication. Furniture is minimal: a bed, a few foot lockers for storage (preferably metal to keep out the rats!) and a plastic table and chairs for daily outdoor dining.*

*A small solar power system is a terrific asset. The combination of panel, battery & an 11-watt bulb provides light at night – great for reading & seeing where the scorpions are hiding! An inverter will produce AC for a computer, which is useful for preparing teaching lessons. By the way, when we say "AC" we mean 'Alternate Current', not 'Air Conditioning'! The latter would certainly be lovely in the searing heat of Sudan... the tents can be comfortable in the middle of the night but definitely not so in the daytime.*

**SIM is committed to living and working among the Sudanese.** *Whether a house is made from mud or block or canvas, SIM missionaries know that what is most needed to live and work in Sudan is **a calling from God & a sincere love for His people.***

---

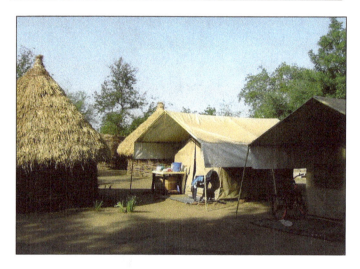

This was my safari tent from January to April 26, 2008, when I left for furlough. It was hot season, and I did not sleep well those sweltering nights. My new tukul was being built. Vicki's and my kitchen tukul is there on the left, sort of in front of my tent.

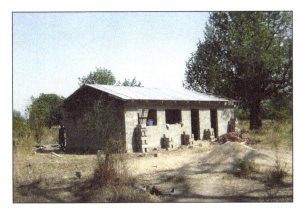

This is our Village Health Worker office and classroom being built with cement blocks in 2007. The student living compound went up behind the classroom.

Meet John Maruti, our friend and Kenyan builder, who built our classroom and many other buildings at Doro.

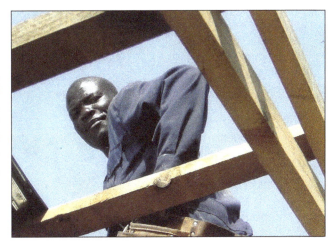

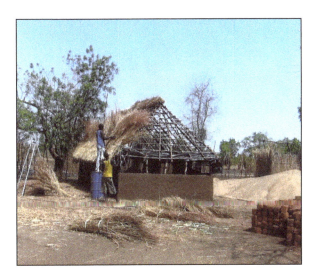

My tukul being built in early 2008. It did not get finished before I left in April for furlough, but I lived there in 2009 and 2010. It is one room with a verandah in front. The entrance was right there where the local builder is standing on the blue barrel.

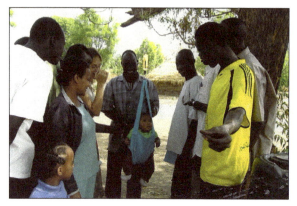

The students are weighing a baby with a hanging scale, tied to a tree limb, on a community outreach day.

Vicki Beattie went with me to help supervise the students.

In 2009 we gave a mosquito net to each mother who came to our well baby clinic. Hundreds of mothers received a net. We taught about malaria and prevention of mosquito bites as our lesson to the gathered mothers.

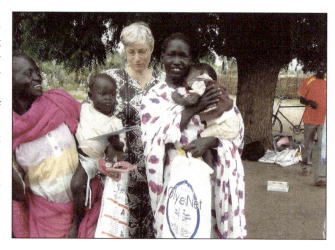

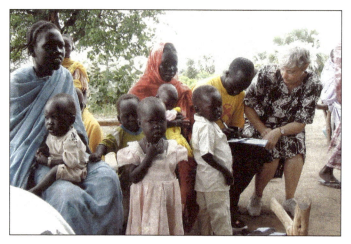

I am teaching a student on community outreach day.

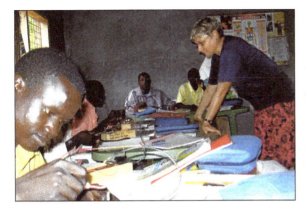

I am teaching inside our classroom.

This happens to be the day we learned about the snake bite shockers as first aid treatment for snake bites and scorpion bites.

We invited the neighborhood children to our classroom to practice head-to-toe exams.

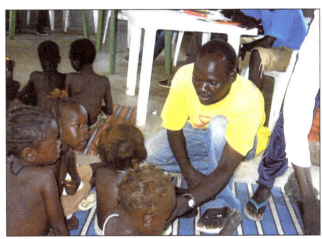

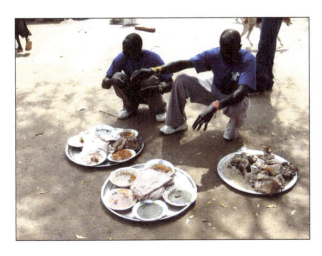

This picture is of our graduation feast with goat meat and kissera, enjoyed by all in the student compound after the graduation program. It really is good food. They served it on big trays for a group of guests to share together.

## Good Practice for Students - Barb Hartwig

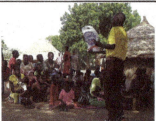

Community Health Worker training is in classroom, community and clinic. We recently completed the first three of nine months of training which has been all about community-based health care thus far. All ten students traveled with us in a wagon pulled by a John Deere tractor along the muddy road to the growing community of Gasmalla. There we split ourselves into three teams . The students started with a devotion followed by health teaching about the use of bednets. Although we brought 200 mosquito nets, there were not enough for every mother who came. As one student summarized our visit, "*We measured children under five, and checked pregnancy mothers. We had gave them some mosquito bednet and weighing them and visiting pregnant mothers. They were very happy with the visit.*" Another student wrote, "*I checked 10 pregnant mothers and 19 children and we gave them mosquito net. And what I learn there, weighing children, hearing babies inside the womb of the mom, giving some medicine to prevent the malaria in pregnant mother.*" Although the "road" is already muddy, we hope to return regularly to follow up weighing babies in the next six months. Now that was a worthwhile day of learning and serving!!

These articles were in our Medical Team Progress Notes

publications of 2009.

## 'Flies with Fingers' - Barb Hartwig

January 28th, 2008 was a landmark day for Vicki Beattie, Dr. Rob Congdon and for me as we opened the Training Center at Doro for the community health workers. Community Health Worker training is a nine month government of South Sudan program with emphasis on community based health care. Health promotion and prevention are as important as medicines.

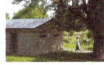

Our twelve Sudanese students are struggling to learn in simple English, but they are doing it! For example, one test question was to write a sanitation "story" about how sicknesses move. I quote one Uduk student's answer, "*Flies, feces, fingers and food are 4 words that start with F. This means flies carrying feces in its finger and put on food. If you eat this food you get diarrhea through fly.*"

Since I am about to leave on furlough (May-December), Vicki bears the load of teaching in the next several months. We had two others lined up to come and help Vicki, but they could not follow through. The workers are few in South Sudan. It is a difficult context to live and work in. Please join us in praying for more willing workers while the peace treaty extends to 2011.

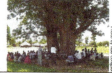

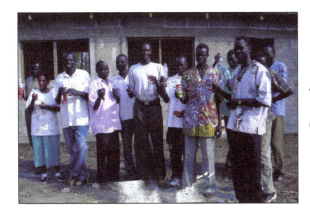

Village Health Workers

Class of 2008

Village Health Workers

Class of 2009

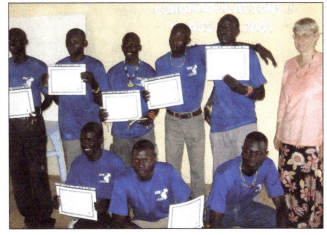

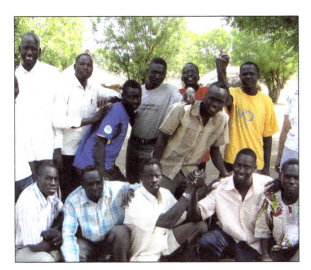

Village Health Workers

Class of 2010

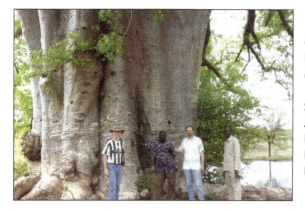

Gotta show you this huge baobab tree near the clinic at Doro.

Standing are:
Jimmy Cox
Pastor Andrew Kena
Dr. Rob Congdon
Daniel Yohr, evangelist

Four of us missionary ladies relaxing after an evening meal:

Abebech (Ethiopian)
Sandy Ewan
Vicki Beattie
myself

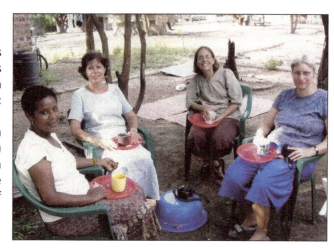

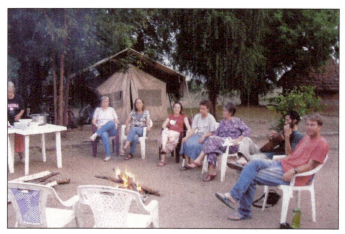

This was taken on my last evening at Doro, my farewell dinner.

November 2010.

212

**20/10/2010**

**TO ALL AGENCIES/DEVELOPMENTAL PARTNERS**
**SOUTHERN SUDAN**

**TRAINING OF COMMUNTY AND MATERNAL HEALTH WORKERS ON HOLD**

The Ministry of Health, Government of Southern Sudan is concerned about the continuous training of Community Health Workers (CHWs) and Maternal and Child Health Workers (MCHWs) despite the existing big number already trained. With the worst health indicators in Southern Sudan and the need to reduce the mortality rates, there is great demand for qualified and skillful Human Resources, including the need to improve the capacity and upgrade the level of the existing Health Care Workers. There is no doubt that training of Nurses and Midwives still remain among the most important priorities of the Ministry. Following the recently concluded assessment on the Health Training Institutions in Southern Sudan, there is also urgent need to embark on improving the standards of these Institutions.

The Ministry of Health is currently reviewing its training priorities; hence request all agencies and developmental partners planning to train CHWs and MCHWs to put it on hold till further notice. The Ministry plans to conduct Ministerial Forum on Human Resource Development (mid next month-Nov) that will give a clear picture and road map of the training priorities of the Government across the 10 states of Southern Sudan.

Thanks for understanding and please note that your continued support is highly appreciated.

**Sincerely,**

**Dr. Olivia Lomoro**
**Under Secretary**
**Ministry of Health**
**Government of Southern Sudan**

CC: Ag. Director General, Human Resource Development
CC: Director General, Nursing and Midwifery

# Part Six

## Assignment: United States

**2011 through February 28, 2013**

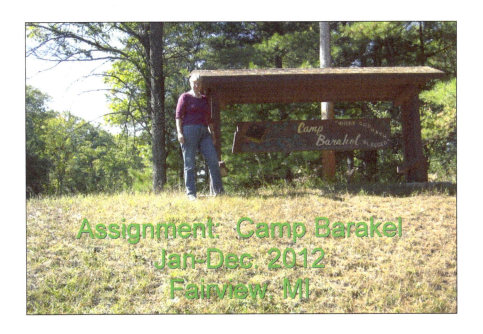

Assignment: Camp Barakel
Jan-Dec, 2012
Fairview, MI

## CHAPTER 18

# WINDING DOWN ON ASSIGNMENT IN THE USA (2011–2012)

*On December 1,* 2010, I arrived home from Africa via Kenya/ South Sudan. I knew that God was leading me to continue with SIM for two more years stateside, and I was praying for clear direction about returning to Africa or not after that. South Sudan was going to finish its comprehensive peace agreement with the North (Khartoum) in 2011 and be declared an independent country. No one knew how smoothly that would pan out, and I was quite content to let them sort their political process out while absent from the country. One thing I had learned from Liberia was that it is one thing to be suddenly caught in a crisis and quite another to be knowingly present when a crisis is likely to occur.

God led me to follow the desire of my heart to prepare to work full-time at a Christian camp in 2012. I began to search for the exact camp in 2011. After a few months of staff nursing at our SIM retirement village in Sebring, Florida, in early 2011, I finally got to go home. From May to December of 2011, I was on furlough (called home assignment). What a wonderful seven months it was. I loved being home. For the first time I lived in the house I grew up in, on the farm by myself (with both parents now in heaven) and could integrate my things, which had been stored away upstairs, into the whole house. Much in the house is the same as when Mom and Dad left. I miss them, but I inherited the house and enjoyed getting it and the yard back into shape after some years of it being unoccupied.

Camp Barakel in Fairview, Michigan, accepted me onto their seasonal staff for one year. Praise the Lord. This is the camp I attended once as a child. My home church was very familiar with this camp. I would remain on SIM support and was technically seconded from SIM to ministry with Camp Barakel, which is about three hours north of Hadley. At camp I was given a cozy, small, furnished, cabin-in-the-woods in which to live. I arrived on January 1, 2012, as they were just starting their winter retreat season the coming weekend. At first I was assigned to help the registrar in the office. I was concerned about the cold winter and how I would adjust after so many years in the hot African climate. I had not spent a whole winter in Michigan since 1981–82! I was glad for all the cold weather clothes I had bought. I needed all of them. Having a mattress heating pad on my bed in the cabin was very helpful on cold winter nights. After a couple of months of office work, I went on to assist the Trading Post manager as she purchased and organized lots of items that would be for sale all summer. That was fun!

Camp Barakel is an outdoor camp with four seasons of programming. All staff had individual cleaning assignments to do each week. Kathy Curtis and I cleaned Snowshoe Lodge every week. Cleaning is not my favorite job, but at Barakel I learned more about doing it, and it turned out to not be so bad after all. In the summer I worked every day in the "medicine cabin," which was the nursing office. Of course, I was responsible for first aid, medicine distribution to campers and staff, and was on call, etc. It was a privilege to choose a missions project from Senegal for the summer campers to contribute to and to present that project each week at chapel. Fall retreats were a combination of teen groups, women's groups, and men's groups. I also did a lot of kitchen work at camp. Every Wednesday morning the staff ladies baked dozens of homemade cookies for the weekend. My days were filled with behind-the-scenes work and I loved it, but I usually went home for my day and a half off each week. This homesick feeling that had started toward the end of my time at Doro was only getting worse. I just wanted to go home and stay. By August of 2012 my decision was made with God's inner peace to not return to Africa, but to resign from SIM in February of 2013. That month would mark thirty years of missionary work and ministry.

First I told my family, close friends, and home church of my final decision not to return to Africa. I told the mission leaders I would resign. Then I wrote a special letter informing my faithful supporters, and finally, I wrote my last prayer letter, which went out to almost 500 people and is included at the end of this chapter. I should have gone to each of my supporting churches and told them in person, but

I knew that I would only have tears and find it emotionally difficult to explain in a service. Please forgive me, dear friends and churches, for not saying thank you and farewell in person to all. Good-byes have always been difficult for me to do without tears.

Before I close these memoirs, I want to say a word about being single. God has truly given me the gift of celibacy. I know very well that I could not have done even half of what I did if I had married. Remaining single for the sake of the kingdom of heaven, to dedicate myself to serving God, is not a sacrifice to me. I have not been lonely. I am content to be single and am able to live on my own, for God has given me all I need and more as I keep trusting in Him.

The idea of never marrying or having children is almost inconceivable in the African culture. There was pressure on me by some national people to marry, and a lot of offers too! Oh, yes. I learned not to wear any rings in Africa. No matter what finger I might put a ring on, they would take it to be marriage. And I did not want to deceive anyone, as I saw some single missionaries try to do. Nor did I want to continually have to explain when someone assumed I had a husband somewhere because I had a ring on. I had an answer ready for any national who asked me why I was not married. I said, "If God gives me a husband, I will marry. But up to now, God has not given me a husband, and I can serve God with all of my time." This seemed to satisfy most Christians. It was important not to say I did not want to marry, or would not marry. I would, and I will, marry if God gives me the right man to love. In First Corinthians, chapter seven, God clearly indicates that He does not expect everyone to marry. Paul wrote this to those unmarried: "not to restrict you, but that you may live in a right way in undivided devotion to the Lord."

Besides those few words about being single, let me add some thoughts about women in ministry. A lot of what I did in Africa was teaching, which was mostly Bible and health. Topics like being a wife and mother were ones I avoided. Being a nurse, however, gave me a platform for many subjects upon which I could advise. On my missionary prayer card is a short version of Luke 9:2-and He sent them to preach the kingdom of God and to heal the sick. I have never preached a sermon, but I did a lot of teaching. Not preaching, which was not for lack of opportunity in Africa, but because I personally do not interpret Scripture as allowing women to be in the position of pastoral leadership. What I do see in Scripture are many examples of women in teaching roles. There is no distinction of male or female in Galatians 3:28 regarding salvation, gifts, and graces. Women are included in the commission of world evangelization in Acts 2:17–18. Philip the evangelist had four daughters who were prophetesses (Acts 21:9). The kind of teaching I did was not domineering. Often it was the national pastor who asked me to teach, and he was my interpreter and added his own commentary to my words. I know that the Holy Spirit within me would have pricked my conscience if I was doing wrong to teach both men and women. Suffice it to say, I often did teach men and mixed groups when invited, and the Lord did work through such opportunities. Actually, I am on the conservative side of women in ministry. I know that some reading this will not agree. After studying Scripture as a whole on this subject, not just one or two verses, this is how the Spirit led me to understand this sometimes controversial subject of women in ministry and teaching mixed groups of men and women.

I do not have many regrets for the thirty years of missionary work that I was privileged to be a part of. Yes, I regret certain words I said or something I did that was wrong at the time. Writing these memoirs has caused me to do some deep soul searching and led me to pray for forgiveness in some cases in which I found I still harbored hurt feelings. The hard things like having to leave a place before I wanted to, dangerous situations, three missionary deaths, and some tough national church/mission relationships could have made me leave missionary work sooner, but God gave me the spiritual faith and perseverance to learn lessons and carry on. Balancing out the tough things is remembering the kids at schools and churches where I got to teach, the village health volunteers, the traditional midwives meetings, refugee camp work, Bible lessons with men and women, and all the good friends I have made among missionaries scattered all over the world. First Corinthians 15:58 says, "Therefore, my beloved brethren, be steadfast, immovable, always abounding in the work of the Lord, knowing that your toil is not in vain in the Lord." Whether overseas, or across the street, let us labor and know that our lives proclaim Christ whether in word or deed or our very presence.

In all the countries I worked in, the church services usually ended by the congregation reciting the last verse of the book of 2 Corinthians. Many times we would go outside the church and stand in a circle of unity and love, holding hands, reciting together: "The grace of the Lord Jesus Christ, and the love of God, and the fellowship of the Holy Spirit, be with you all." Amen.

*'Tis So Sweet to Trust in Jesus*

by Louisa M. R. Stead, 1882

'Tis so sweet to trust in Jesus, Just to take Him at His word;
Just to rest upon His promise; Just to know, "Thus saith the Lord."
Jesus, Jesus, how I trust Him!
How I've proved Him o're and o're!
Jesus, Jesus, precious Jesus!
O for grace to trust Him more!
I'm so glad I learned to trust Thee, Precious Jesus, Savior, Friend;
And I know that Thou art with me, Wilt be with me to the end.

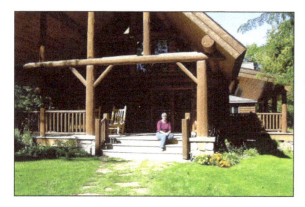

This is Camp Barakel's office building. It is a beautiful, rustic wood structure.

At one winter retreat my niece and nephew, Tyler and Briana, were at Camp, and we had fun tubing downhill.

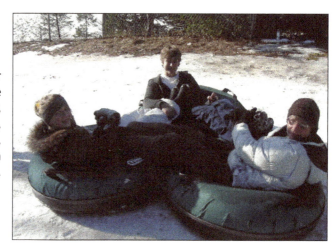

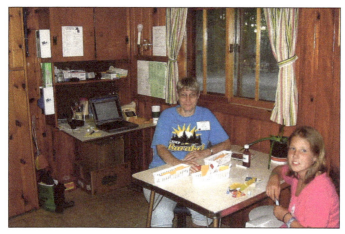

I worked in the "medicine cabin" all summer. I got to know some campers and counselors very well.

## This is my final prayer letter.

Serving with
SIM
Box 7900
Charlotte, NC 28241

December 2012
(my name and contact information were here)

Dear family and friends,

In February of 1983 I took a big step of faith when I left New York City shores in a big plane for my first assignment in Africa. I loved those nine years in Liberia, teaching Bible and health. Then the civil war in Liberia shifted me over to Ethiopia for a temporary assignment which lasted 4 years. What with Liberia still unstable in 1997, I took an assignment in northern Ghana that would fulfill my dream of being on a church planting team plus starting a community-based health care program from scratch out in about 15 villages. What fun to educate and enable village volunteers to promote good health habits while teaching Bible in churches.

Then came one day in January 2005 when I heard on BBC radio that north and south Sudan signed a peace agreement. Hurrah for the southern people! I knew SIM would re-enter south Sudan with a development team and I wanted to be part of it. I transferred from Ghana to South Sudan in January 2006 and began five years of what was probably the best work I have done. My previous experience enabled me to start up, lead and teach health workers for rural clinics. Now that program has been suspended by the government of South Sudan in lieu of desiring the training of three year nurses.

South Sudan declared independence from northern Sudan in July 2011. As about 90,000 displaced people moved into the county around Doro due to border and oil disputes, I stayed stateside in 2011 and 2012. Thank you Camp Barakel director, Paul Gardner, and staff for the privilege of working with you this year in northern Michigan while I continued to watch, wait and pray about my next move.

The decision I have faced is whether to return to South Sudan or stay in Hadley, Michigan. I have declined to start over in a new country in Africa again which would require some language learning. After much prayerful consideration I have decided to stay home in Hadley. I would like to go back to South Sudan someday to hand over the training program at Doro to someone else should the opportunity arise.

This situation coincides with my 30 year mark as an active member of SIM. As of February 28th, 2013 I will resign from SIM. I am not eligible by age yet to retire from SIM and get the housing allowance that should be there for me when I do request reinstatement for retirement from SIM in about 10 years.

How does one begin to say **Thank You** to the churches and individuals who have prayed, given support, love, packages and encouragement to me these many years?? My home church, Hadley Community Church, who commissioned me to go to Africa in 1983, has faithfully supported me at 50% of whatever amount of support was required all of these years. So many others also supported me the whole 30 years and I thank you very much. My family has been behind me the whole time and I thank them for the sacrifices they made to give me their blessing. Most of all, I thank God, our Lord and Savior, for the privilege of serving Him in Sub-Sahara Africa. They certainly go down as the best years of my life. The real impact of that service is immeasurable in numbers and will only be known one glad day of reunion in heaven! He brought me out of four situations that were extremely dangerous, only to strengthen my resolve to continue. Certainly at Christmas time when we sing about His name Immanuel it should be a stark reminder of God with us through thick and thin. Surely each of us has a story to tell of God's provision, God's perfect timing, and God's faithfulness.

Thank you again and may your Christmas Season be blessed beyond measure!

Yours sincerely in the Hope and Promise of eternal life
through Jesus Christ our Lord, Amen. *Bert*

Printed in the USA
CPSIA information can be obtained
at www.ICGtesting.com
JSHW011103141123
52031JS00001B/2